# WEIGHT TRAINING

---

## A BEGINNERS GUIDE TO BUILDING A LEANER, BIGGER, STRONGER BODY, NATURALLY AND EASILY

### VINCE KOWALSKI

# CONTENTS

# INTRODUCTION

"What is the point of being on this Earth if you are going to be like everyone else?"

- ***Arnold Schwarzenegger***

I'm really glad you're here, because the quicker you learn what the right ways and the wrong ways are, the quicker you'll be just that bit closer to your dream body. That inspirational destination. And that's why we're here, right? Awesome.

Thankfully, you won't have to learn through mistakes; because I've already done them for you! Yep, tried and tested right here. In fact, I never had anyone teach me, but through trial and error, I've come up with a pretty good understanding of the art of building a body.

Hi! My name is Vince Kowalski, and I'm a polish-born American from California. I'm 28 years old and I've got 10 years of training behind me. I don't hold a personal trainer's degree, however, my opinion on those degrees is that... most of the time, they don't hold much merit, anyway. I mean, there are so many courses that go for 6 months then "BAM!" You can go and train someone? Without even obtaining the results yourself? I mean, let's be real, the greatest body-builder of all time is Schwarzenegger, and he didn't hold a personal trainer's licence. But, I bet you would take his advice, right? Yes! Because he's been through it, he's done it, and so he knows what it takes to get it.

So, that's what this whole title is about. I want to share my experience with you. And so, you don't have to make the same mistakes as I did, and you can jumpstart your bodybuilding goals with real form. Whether you want to lose weight or gain weight, there is information here for anyone, female or male, and any body type. I will share with you the science behind muscle gain, the different body types, high protein recipes, training schedules for beginners, and well, a hell of a lot more, too! Thanks for joining me here. I know you'll get the most out of it. And I know you can start right away, after you've finished reading this. Let's go!

# 1

---

## MUSCLE SCIENCE

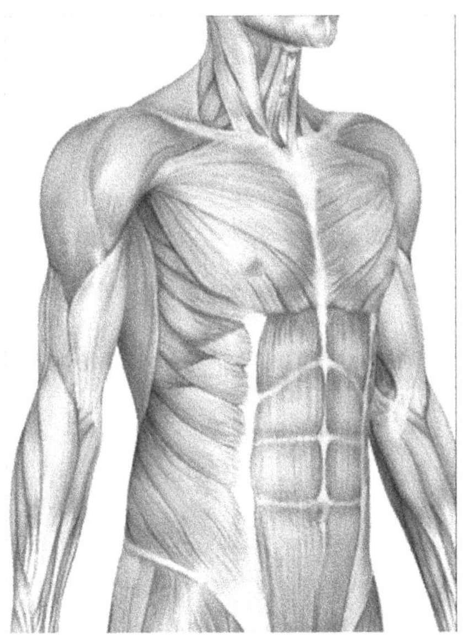

THE BASIC SCIENCE OF MUSCLE GROWTH IS IMPORTANT IN weight training. When you understand what muscles need to stay in a state of wellbeing (or homeostasis), then you can aid the preparation and the long-term health of them, as an ongoing key factor. Generally speaking, muscles are adapting to environmental stress, all of the time. And just as the sun tans the body as a defence against burning, the muscles also grow in response of increased stresses built up in the muscles.

Before getting started, we need to take a look at some of the key points and get a clearer picture of why muscles behave in the ways they do:

After you have completed a workout, your body goes through a stage of repairing and replacing damaged muscle fibers. This cellular process is where fibers are fused together and go on to create new muscle myofibrils (protein strands). These myofibrils that have been repaired, they now go on to achieve an increase in thickness and number. This is scientifically what we know as "muscle hypertrophy growth." Muscles grow when there is a rate of muscle protein synthesis, which is more significant than any rate of muscle protein which has broken down.

None of this actually happens while you are lifting the weights. This occurs during your times of rest. You might even begin to wonder; how can I truly add muscle to my muscle cells? Well, this is the function of satellite cells which act like stem cells, although, they are only for your muscles. Once these are activated, they aid by adding more nuclei to your muscle cells and consequently, they then provide direct growth of muscle cells (myofibrils).

It is the activation of satellite cells which might be the difference between how certain "genetic freaks" can grow immense muscles, and why it other people "the hard-gainers" struggle.

Researchers showed that, in a recent study, people who were known as the "extreme" responders toward muscle growth, and had 58% myofibril hypertrophy from working out, actually possessed a 23%

activation of their satellite cells. Compare this to the modest responders, who showed a 28% growth, and who had a 19% activation within their satellite cells.

Even though both of these groups showed an increase, the exciting part was where the "none" responders were placed. They were found to have 0% growth, while having a 0% activation of their satellite cells.

This leads us to believe that: the more you can activate your satellite cells, the better chance you have of being able to grow muscle. Now the question is; how can we activate the satellite cells and encourage muscle growth at the same time?

## Muscle Growing Mechanisms

A natural progression of muscle growth is our capacity to continually keep stressing the muscles. It is this stress that becomes a significant component of muscle growth and it interrupts homeostasis inside your body. This constant stress (and the following interruption of homeostasis) instigates three primary mechanisms that encourage muscle growth.

### 1. Muscular Tension

For us to increase muscle growth, there is a need to apply factors of stress which are higher than what the body (or the muscle) has subsequently become adapted to.

How is this possible? One way to do this; is by lifting weights which are progressively heavier. This places additional tension on the muscles and aids the changes at a cellular level within the tissue. This then allows growth factors which include activation of mTOR and the all-important satellite cells.

Muscular tension can also noticeably effect connection of the motor units within the muscle cells. These other two factors can explain why there are stronger people, although they are usually not as large as others.

## 2. Muscular Damage

Muscle damage manifests itself when you feel sore after a workout. This (more often than not) occurs in a specific or localized region. When this happens, inflammatory molecules are released (pain) and immune system cells which activate your satellite cells then jump into action (growth).

This might lead you to think that you have to feel sore in order for this to happen, although, this is not the case. Instead, the damage from the workout needs to be present in your muscle cells. The soreness, on the other hand, is associated with other factors over time.

## 3. Metabolic Stress

You can quickly feel metabolic stress when you "feel the burn" in the gym, or you have had the "pump." Previously, scientists questioned the theory of the pump, however, after further investigation, it appears they are actually onto something.

Swelling around the muscle is caused by metabolic stress which helps with the muscle growth. It doesn't, however, necessarily give an increase in muscle cell size. This actually occurs when there is an increase in muscle glycogen, which swells the muscles at the same time as the connective tissues grow. This type of growth has been termed "sarcoplasmic hypertrophy," and is one of the primary ways individuals appear to have more extensive muscles without an increase in their strength to match it.

Now we can understand the three primary factors which lead to muscle growth, and our next question is: how will our hormones affect muscle growth? Let's look at that next.

Muscle Growth and Hormones

Hormones also play an essential role in muscle growth and repair, and this is due to their role in the regulation of satellite cell activity. Insulin Growth Factor (IGF)-1 and (especially) Mecho-Growth Factor (MGF) are needed, both of these (along with testosterone) are two of the most crucial operators that promote muscle growth.

When working out, testosterone is what most people associate with being the primary hormone. There does come some validity in the thought. Actually yes; testosterone aids in increasing protein synthesis, activating the satellite cells, inhibiting protein breakdown, as well as stimulating various other anabolic hormones.

In truth, the majority of testosterone is bound to the body, and consequently not accessible to use (up to 98%). And signs that strength training aids in not only releasing higher levels of testosterone, but similarly making the muscle cells more sensitive to any free testosterone, is definitely true.

Testosterone also aids in stimulating responses of growth hormone. This is performed by the increase in the presence of neurotransmitters in the damaged fiber region. This can also help in the activation of tissue growth.

The IGF adjusts the amounts of muscle-mass growth, doing this by boosting any protein synthesis. This is done by facilitating the body's glucose acceptance and the repartitioning of amino acids (amino acids are the building blocks of protein). This repartitioning allows the skeletal muscle structure, and again, helps in activating the satellite cells which lead to an increase in muscle growth, overall.

**The Need for Muscle Rest to Be Able to Grow**

If the body is not given sufficient nutrition or rest, the anabolic processes can be reversed, and the body will fall into a catabolic or destructive state.

Muscle protein metabolism responses happen (from resistance exercises), and they last between 24-48 hours. Therefore, interactions between meals consumed in this period and any protein metabolism are linked.

It is worth keeping in mind, limitations are in place of how much your muscles can physically grow. Much of which is dependent on gender, age, and genetics. As a prime example, male bodies have more testosterone than that of females, which will allow them to build larger and stronger muscle groups, overall.

## Unlikely & Rapid Muscle Growth

Muscle growth for the majority of people is slow, and this is because muscle hypertrophy takes time. Most people will not see any visible increase for several weeks, or in some cases, months. This is due to the ability of how well your nervous system activates your muscles.

Secondary to this, and uniquely, people have different genetics. These variances in hormonal output, muscle fiber types, and physical numbers make a difference. Satellite cell activation levels can also restrict muscle growth.

To ensure you're doing your best to grow muscle, muscle protein synthesis must exceed your muscle protein breakdown. This helps to make sure you are performing at your best to, infact, build muscle. This necessitates that you consume adequate sources of protein (specifically essential amino acids) and carbohydrates too, which aid the cellular process when rebuilding any broken-down muscle tissues.

It is essential for you to understand the science behind what enables muscles to grow, because any visible muscle growth and apparent physical changes in the muscle structure of your body, can be extremely encouraging.

2

———

# POSITIVE MINDSETS

"Vision creates faith and faith creates willpower. With faith there is no anxiety and no doubt - just absolute confidence in yourself."

**- *Arnold Schwarzenegger***

The previous bodybuilding champions of our generations came to rely on numerous strategies; ones which enabled them to power their way through grueling workouts. This led them to achieve the physiques which continually inspire all newcomers to the sport of today.

Training and diet are the two primary aspects which are associated with the achievement of reaching physical perfection. However, there is another, more fundamental variable, which has aided champions like Schwarzenegger, Haney, and Coleman, to name just a few. This is the concept of mind power, or their belief in themselves.

When you possess the ability to connect on a psychological level with your muscles, then using various strategies can be crucial for success. Arnold Schwarzenegger saw (and convinced himself) his biceps would grow to become mountain peaks. It has to be said, he achieved some amazing, and what some would claim, "unparalleled muscle development" in this area.

Another was Tom Platz, who envisaged his quads becoming like giant balloons. Have you seen anyone who can rival his leg development? There is something to be said about mindset here, and that if you imagine the unthinkable, you might reach tremendous gains. However, using mind power in aiding your bodybuilding accomplishments can be significantly more complicated. It takes real focus and determination.

## Mind Focus

Overall, mental focus takes immense effort if complete concentration is sought after. When you are trying to complete any set with necessary intensity, attention to correct your form (while still maintaining visualization) takes complete focus.

One of the best strategies for improving your focus, is to sit quietly before each set while considering the tasks you have set yourself. And this should be done as a way of blocking out all unnecessary information.

Stray conversations, the radio, or any off-putting thoughts and/or people who are in your direct vicinity need to go. These can all be seen as interruptions and are of no use as far as your perfect set is concerned.

It is also useful to map out exactly what you wish to achieve for any specific set. This includes the number of repetitions, a correct form, and the feeling in your muscles. These distinctions all qualify as significant factors, and they are very worthy of your attention.

## Preserving a Positive Mindset

Positive visualizations and setting goals are crucial variables when pursuing the improvement of one's mindset. In fact, maintaining your focus is, without a doubt, very important, as was illustrated in the previous section. It is, however, equally as important to uphold an affirmative mindset all of the time. This is true, even when you're not training.

Many social problems are all around us in today's fast-paced world. It is not always easy to sustain calmness and focus for any substantial period of time. Nevertheless, it is exceptionally desirable to attempt and develop a positive mindset. Top professionals in any sport usually possess very few external distractions, and in turn, allowing them the satisfaction of being able to concentrate on training objectives with relative efficiency.

The secret while performing any physical event (weight training included) is to mentally place yourself in a moment where you are at the highest possible level. Being preoccupied with yesterday's occurrences, or what could happen tomorrow are irrelevant to the task at hand, and should be blocked from your thoughts, altogether.

When you can maintain a positive mindset, it is much easier to switch off and submerge yourself in your training regime. When you focus on any negative qualities of life, this only dilutes what is happening within the present time, and as a result, you will find it impedes your training performance.

There are various ways you can enhance your positive thinking, and these include, distancing yourself from negative people, or refraining from undesirable activities such as laziness, excessive alcohol use, or smoking.

Positive visualizations and the setting of goals are important factors when looking to improve your positive mindset. In the moments you sit quietly before each set, envisage precisely what you want achieved during your set. This can be done in the hour before each training session and has been shown to offer great value.

On the other hand, if you think about your workout 24-hours-per-day, it is not very conducive to the development of a positive mindset. This can (and is more likely to) lead to mental burnout and discouragement.

## The Mind & Body Link

For you to achieve complete mental focus, it is essential for you to develop your mind and muscle links. It has been proven; the more superior the aptitude an athlete has in their chosen sport, the more they become more skillful at using a particular action or specific exercise. This is true, especially when they can precisely target particular muscle groups.

Undeniably, and as far as bodybuilding goes, it is vital to visualize the influence accurately. This is for what effect any particular exercise is having on specific muscles. The better a person becomes at this, the better they can successfully develop their mind and muscle links.

What is the best way to achieve this? When you study all of your different muscle groups and acquire the ability in identifying the individual muscles, you can eventually come to learn to know if these exercises have the desired effect. Then, you will do it intuitively, without conscious thought.

Many people can lift a weight for a predetermined number of repetitions. However, very few are aware of the mind and muscle links, and precisely how this weight training is assisting in their overall muscle growth.

Arnold Schwarzenegger recommended the flexing of body parts before training them. He called this; "Getting in touch with your muscles." This is a simple way in which to develop the mind and muscle links.

A good example is flexing the chest by pushing the arms out. This replicates the actions you will perform on a bench press. It is this pushing action that leads the mind to know precisely how the bench press exercise should feel. When you perform the bench press, more fibers will be activated as the lifting motion has been put in the groove, this happens through the pre-flexing of the muscles.

Another way of enforcing your mind and muscle links is to have a training partner casually touch the area which you are going to train. You will find your attention is subconsciously directed toward this area, and, as a result, training energies will become more focused and in line with how you will perform the exercise.

When you have strengthened the mind and muscle links, you can also negate muscular restrictions. This acts in a similar way to a warmup, and it also stretches the desired muscles which help to prevent muscle damage from the heavy lifting. A good example being heavy squats, where severe exertion is placed on the muscles.

## Subconscious Conditioning

The goal of being able to gain vast amounts of muscle will take more than purely psyching yourself up for your training session... and blocking out any distractions. These things can be significant, although, to achieve an element of outstanding success, you must condition your subconscious mind. Your subconscious is the region of the mind which operates just under the level of your awareness.

Everything in life, be it real or imaginary, can stimulate you on a subconscious level, and therefore, lead you to think or act in very specific ways. To sum it up: negative thinkers tend to encounter adverse events. While, on the other hand, people who continually think positively, they tend to obtain the most out of life.

The real champions in bodybuilding rarely speak of themselves in a negative light, and always paint themselves in a positive light. This is done on purpose. Additionally, they are inclined to be equally positive in most areas of their life.

When you aim to become (and remain) an eternal optimist, it can change your entire life. This can quite-possibly be the single, most significant step a champion can make. In fact, the best way to condition your subconscious, is to practice positive affirmations on a continual basis.

Affirmations are positive thoughts or statements which you repeat to yourself. These become implanted in your subconscious as a foundation of inspiration for present and future actions. Affirmations can teach the subconscious to overpower mental and physical barriers, ones which were previously thought impossible. These are one of the easiest and best tools for overcoming negative thought processes, and they go a long way to enhancing your self-esteem as an individual.

## Awesome Bodybuilding Affirmations

*"I will have the power for today's workout and I will overwhelm any barriers."*

*"I will exceed all my personal bests, today."*

*"The healthy foods I eat will contribute to my superior muscle growth."*

These affirmations are a respectable start, but, it is best to select them on a specific basis for predetermined goals. An affirmation which is too broad will never work, this is because you will not have a particular goal focus in mind.

Trigger words can be used to personally motivate and stimulate you.

A trigger word could be "spectacular," for example. As in, "I will experience spectacular results today." Use words which stimulate and excite you. Do them in the mirror every morning and evening to train your subconscious mind.

## Setting Goals

Setting goals is conductive to your success when weight training and they will also help you to maximize your results. The one main thing you have to decide on is, what are you looking to actually achieve by setting these goals? This gives meaning to the goals you set for yourself.

Both long-term and short-term goals should be set. Short term goals should cover 1 week up to 6 months, and long-term should cover 6 months and over.

A good rule to follow is setting three short-term goals that equate to one long-term goal.

## Short-Term Goals

Example:

Use every piece of gym equipment available and perform one set within the first two weeks of training.

Performing sit-ups for 3 sets consisting of 12 reps on all abdominal days.

Replace one meal during the day with a salad or supplement.

## Long-Term Goals

Example:

Aim to lose 40 pounds in 8 months.

Within 1 year be able to bench press 160 pounds.

Within 6 months increase bicep size to 14 inches.

## Keys of Effective Affirmation Usage

- Use affirmations which are specific to your goals
- Start every day with a positive affirmation
- Use affirmations frequently (say them to yourself throughout the day)
- Use only positive words, and replace negative ones with a positive alternative
- Act like your affirmations are working

Mind training, as described in this chapter, is as essential as any muscle training when you are aiming for superior results. When you read anything about previous bodybuilding champions, all this becomes apparent.

When it comes to your motivation, anyone can condition their mind for greatness. A well-conditioned mind is half the battle in building muscle; if you can picture it, you can do it.

The conditioning of your mind for greatness though, is not a simple process. You need to perform plenty of planning and effort. Through the focusing of your mind and being able to attain and maintain your positive mindset, you can do anything. And, with the strengthening of your mind and muscle links, this is a wonderful preparation. Healthy conditioning of the subconscious can lead you toward incredible results. Start now; and think your way to having a great physique.

"The mind is the limit. As long as the mind can envision the fact that you can do something, you can do it, as long as you really believe 100 percent."

**- *Arnold Schwarzenegger***

3

———————

# THREE PILLARS

LET'S TAKE A LOOK AT THE IMPORTANCE OF THE "THREE Pillars" as a concept for our ongoing focus for successful weight training. When we look at this pivotal strategy, we can gauge the key areas of focus placement, which can, therefore, bring about success, growth, and health maintenance that is safe, result-based and positive in nature. As with any new regime or plan, the importance of health and safety are always the priority. When the three pillars are maintained, the results are more definitive and progressive. Additionally, safety and health will remain at the forefront, and as an ongoing necessity in the weight training goal.

With a complete focus on the three pillars, you can consistently bring great results, over time. And, in reality, the need for great results is the purpose of weight training, for us to meet our end goal/s.

The 3 Pillars Are:

- Sleep

- Training
- Nutrition


## **Metaphorically Speaking: Homeostasis**

Let's think outside the box, just for a moment. Let's use a car. Let's use that as a metaphor here, just so we can get the gist of the important point we're trying to understand. So, basically, you are the car; and you want to be - the best looking, most built piece of work ever made! Don't you? And not just on the outside. You also want the best on the inside, too. The best motor, the best everything, so you roar like a lion not purr like a kitten. And, it doesn't matter what type of car you are... you just want to be the best version of that model; whatever it is.

So, you'll need great fuel (nutrition), great performance mileage (training), and maintained and serviced to keep the car in good shape after all the hell you have put it through(sleep). If any of these things don't get regularly attended too, then you (as the car) will not be a lean machine, all hotted up and raring to go!

It might sound a bit cliché, I suppose, but in reality, we need to look at what works best for the results we're trying to achieve. And you wouldn't put home brand oil in a Nascar, would you? Or forget to let a Lamborghini cool down after it did multiple laps around the circuit? I mean the results wouldn't be achievable, not long term, anyway. Now, even if you don't like cars – that's alright; you can use the same metaphor with a dog, or anything that requires love, care and maintenance. Plants are also an awesome example for the purpose of understanding this concept. I just want you to keep this idea in your mind, so you understand why the three pillars need to be in the forefront of your mind, at all times. Not just sometimes. That way, your health, your performance, your safety, and your work ethic stay aligned to your goals. We want this to occur in a positive, successful mode of ongoing, reality-based achievement. Otherwise, it just won't work.

Let's take river for example: A river has loads of things swimming in it. Fish, and other creatures that rely upon it for their survival. Well, imagine your muscles are fish. Another metaphor, but stay with me, so I can explain...

Okay, so this river needs certain things to make it viable for the fish to thrive and survive. The temperature, the sunshine, the food, the acid/alkalinity level (PH). Yes, they all need to be right, don't they? Well, the "homeostasis" of the river (just like the homeostasis of your body) affects the fish, greatly. So, in essence, if your body is the river, (metaphorically speaking), and your muscles are the "fish," you can see the connection, easily. Your muscles will survive and thrive on the homeostasis of your body. That's certainly true. So, when you make sure the three pillars are maintained, then you too, not only survive, but thrive. And that's the goal here; to give your body the chance to thrive from a weight training perspective.

## Sleep

Sleep and sleep maintenance are important factors in achieving homeostasis for the body. And when the body has ample sleep, it can perform really well. Homeostasis is the "perfect" harmony needed at a cellular level for the body to be performing at its optimal point. The cells can achieve repair, growth and much-needed healing when homeostasis is maintained. That means the cells in the muscles and connective tissue have the chance to grow well, too. Because, as you know, they are made up of cells. And they will also be able to recover more easily and efficiently in a "homeostatic" environment. Treating them right is paramount. It is key.

## Guidelines for Sleep

- 7 to 8 hours per night
- Be in a relaxed state before going to sleep
- Turn off electronic devices 1 to 2 hours before sleep to assist the ease
- Yoga and meditation can aid sleep promotion
- Make the room as dark as possible- sleeping masks are recommend

## Training

- Regular training is key
- Train with a 3-day, split routine
- In weight workouts, focus on compound movements (big muscle groups)
- Focus on the larger muscle groups – upper back, chest, shoulders, calves, thighs, arms, and abdominals
- Positivity is key
- Reward yourself with positive affirmations and stress-free downtime

## Nutrition

- Eat 3 to 5 well-balanced meals each day
- Include "flesh" foods like fish, pork, chicken, beef, eggs, and milk
- Supplement your diet with nutrients, vitamins and minerals from nutritious foods not vitamin tablets

## Balance is Key

To have optimal muscle growth, the three pillars must be in balance. All three are just as are important as each other. A regime where proper sleep and training are undertaken; but where a bad diet is allowed, will not work. In this instance, the muscles will repair slowly, and injuries can occur from unhealed and overworked muscles.

Proper diet and great training without the sleep will see the denotation where the same situation applies. And because the muscles are not rested, therefore, they do not repair and grow.

And lastly, good eating habits with great sleep; in conjunction with a poor training regime, will not work either. In this instance, there will not be the right resistance to the muscles for them to adapt and grow properly.

The three pillars create a homeostatic environment for the cells (and therefore, muscles) to grow, heal, repair and maintain health, for the long term.

Write the three pillars down on your goal board to help you remember the importance of them. This is the most pivotal addition to your success. And remember this key concept can mean the difference between success and failure.

4

---

# BODYBUILDING MYTHS

I think it's super-important to look at the facts and myths surrounding the whole topic surrounding bodybuilding. By doing this, we can do the right things from the get-go. And, I know you work hard for your cash, and so you deserve to spend it on the things that *really* matter, like gym membership, nutritious foods, and supplements that really do work.

In this chapter, I'm going to talk about some extremely popular products that may sound great on paper, but that are actually a waste of your cash.

Sometimes, individuals might react defensively when you tell them that a "savior supplement" they've been using for many years is a total waste of time and money, but remember, I'm giving you my insight to help you, and so you can divert that hard-earned cash into something more useful. Okay, so here we go...

## Protein Powders and Pre-Workouts

Protein powders and health supplements make up a billion-dollar industry, and many businesses wish to be a part of it because of the gain. This can lead to many products being released that either don't do as they say, or they come with potential health risks. That's not good for our purposes and will not accentuate the three pillars as required. We need to utilize that focus, to both sustain and maintain health. We also need it to ensure muscle performance, healing, growth and our long-term success with our end goal/s.

## Dmaa

This is one ingredient that is generally found in pre-workout powders or pills and has many potential health risks associated with it. It can increase your blood pressure and heart rate. Other side effects of DMAA are as follows:

- Seizures
- Heart Palpitations
- Fainting
- Kidney Failure
- Liver Failure
- Cardiac Arrest

## Creatine

This is a natural substance created by the body and can give a boost of energy. It can, though, bring with it side effects such as dehydration, muscle cramps, stomach cramps, diarrhea, and nausea (among others).

Although used by many athletes, they stop using it before a competition because creatine causes fluids to flow into the muscles - which makes them look bigger. The downside is they lose definition and the tissue can feel soft and unnatural.

## Protein Powders

These can be made from soy protein, pea protein and the most common (being whey protein). Although there are some great natural alternatives such as bone broth protein powder, the majority of big name companies' products (when taken for extended periods), can actually have serious health risks.

A research study was conducted which showed certain protein powders were laced with traces of particularly harmful heavy metals. These included cadmium, mercury and arsenic. It is the inclusion of these substances that go a long way to making people feel sick with long-term usage.

A single dose of whey protein of 50 grams or 30 grams per day is well within limits, yet many protein powders contain much higher amounts than the recommended dose. Some go as far as 50 grams and above per serving.

Side effects of whey protein can include, yet are not limited to:

- Abnormal heart rhythms
- Changes in cholesterol levels and increased diabetes risk
- Kidney dysfunction and liver damage
- Stomach problems including: bloating, constipation, cramps, gas, and diarrhea
- Reduced appetite
- Swelling of limbs and movement problems
- Headaches and nausea
- Increased fracture or osteoporosis risk
- An increase in acne

Whey protein can also lower blood sugar levels and can have a significant effect on people with diabetes.

A few people find they also react when using protein powders. A prime example is people who are allergic to milk. As whey is a by-product of making cheese, it is directly related to dairy and will bring the same effects.

When you look at protein powders on the whole, they can be beneficial if you use the right ones. Sometimes, due to the quantities required, they can cause side effects. So, you need to make sure you buy them from a reputable supplier. Then, the correct quantities will be utilized for your body's functionality.

There are also the ingredients which are not listed that can be harmful, mainly if these powders are produced overseas where there are no strict regulations for manufacturing processes. Be discerning for your health. When you buy the right ones, they can be amazingly beneficial and accelerate your results!

## Soy Protein & Hormones

Although not as popular as whey protein, soy protein is used in a good many products. Although a few side effects might be similar to the effects of whey protein, soy-based products have another possible side effect; namely, hormonal disruption.

Soy is rich in amino acids which are essential to the body's function, yet they are also full of phytoestrogen which will mimic the natural estrogen that is found in the body. This can have effects on the body as the endocrine systems become unstable. Added to this, nearly 95% of soy products are genetically modified when they are used in protein powders, and it is the inclusion of ridiculous amounts of glyphosate that leads to this hormonal imbalance.

For women, this may not be as much as a problem as it is for men, because estrogen is more of a "female" hormone. Soy products of this nature (when consumed in large amounts and for long periods) can lead to erectile dysfunction. The libido is lowered, and breasts can start to form in men. This performs much the same way as steroid usage in women occurs. The body is exposed to a change in chemical structure and levels that really mess with the body's functions. Not allowing for homeostasis (or balance).

## Steroids

Steroids are a synthetic compound that tries to mimic the body's own naturally produced testosterone. The purpose of testosterone is to attach itself to a cell and then aid in the synthesis of protein. Although steroids are used for medical conditions, they are heavily monitored and generally only use one steroid at a time.

When used in weight training to improve recovery time and muscle growth, they are used at between ten and one hundred times the prescribed dosage. On many occasions, there is also more than one steroid being used. Due to the strength of these steroids, there are many harmful side effects a person may be challenged with.

## Steroidal Effects on Certain Body Structures:: Brain

Aggressive behavior is one of the significant impacts of high levels of testosterone in the body. This can leave a person feeling euphoric, depressed, and paranoid, and having major mood swings.

**Face**

Steroids retain fluids in the body, and one sign of steroid abuse is a round and puffy face. Women have also been shown to grow facial hair and have a more profound voice than usual.

**Eyes**

If a person uses steroids for extended periods, they can develop significant eyes problems. These can include glaucoma, cataracts and general eye infections.

## Hair

With steroid use, the hair follicles narrow. Now, a user begins to grow hair that is thinner, and after a while, these follicles die which can lead the user to become bald.

## Heart

As steroids increase cholesterol levels, long-term use of steroids can lead to cardiovascular diseases. Blood pressure can rise and can lead to blood clots and finally have to heart or stroke problems.

## Kidneys and Liver

The function of the kidneys is to remove harmful waste from the blood, and to regulate salt and water levels in the body. Oral steroids hinder the role of the kidneys, so they become overworked at trying to clean the blood. With continual use, there are chances that kidney stones can form. As with the liver, this is also used to filter toxins from the blood. Symptoms of liver damage are jaundice which is the yellowing of the skin and the eyes.

## Impotence

As the body receives other sources of testosterone, the natural production ceases. This can make the testicles shrink as they are no longer required. With long-term usage, a user can become impotent and not be able to achieve an erection.

## Overall

These are only a few of the side effects of steroid use, and it is easy to see why they are such a danger to human life.

It is far better to eat healthily with the right supplements and train hard to achieve your goal - without any of the huge risks involved. You will also see that your muscle definition is more balanced and looks more natural than if steroids have been used.

Achieving a great body doesn't need steroids. They are only aiming to replicate the body's natural function, yet much more quickly.


## Some Other Disreputable Mentions:

I won't go into great detail on these, but here's a quick look at other supplements and fillers you should definitely avoid:

- HMB
- D-Ribose
- DHEA
- Methoxy
- Ecdysterone
- Myostatin Inhibitors
- Waxy Maize (including other similar "after workout" carbohydrate powders)
- Chromium Picolinate
- Vanadyl Sulphate
- Low Quality Protein Bars
- Growth Hormone Boosters


## Genetics

A lot of people use their genetics as an excuse not to achieve the body they desire. It should be noted, these are the people who visit the gym once a week or every ten days. It is too easy to blame something else rather than face the real reason. Laziness and lack of motivation are major causes here.

It is true much of our body type does come from our genetics, and we can fall into one of three body types.

**Ectomorphs** are tall and thin and have a low-fat storage capacity. These body types are not known for getting fat and building muscle.

**Mesomorphs** have a medium body type, with low-fat levels and broad shoulders with narrow waists. Often, these are called "muscular" and can build muscle without storing fat.

**Endomorphs** have wide waists and large bone structures. This is what is generalized as fat. They also find it easy to store fat.

## Screw Genetics

Everyone's body burns energy in different ways which are dependent on our body type. This has more than likely been handed down to us on a genetic level, yet it is no excuse for this to stand in your way of achieving the body you want.

Your diet is responsible for 50% to 60% of your success with your training program making up the remaining 20% and sleep another 20%.

To succeed in getting the body you want, you have to adapt your diet and training regime. It might be that you have skinny forearms and calves yet eating correctly and focusing on these areas can change your physique to the one you desire.

Genetics are a part of all of us, and there is no getting away from it. They do not, however, make us the person we want to be. That is something we control ourselves, as long as we change the way we go about it.

I can tell you from experience, that your dream body is very possible. It's up to you to achieve it, and I know you can! With the three pillars and a great help from the right supplements. You are worth every ounce of time.

**Some Training Tidd-Bits to Match Your Body Type**

Do you know if you are you an ectomorph, endomorph, or meso-morph? It's an important question, because the type of body you were born with can have a big impact on how effective your training will be. Especially in the long-term. And, if you know what type you are, then you can target training and develop a workout regime that matches it, and you can get ready for some awesome gains, too!

We all have unique body types. Some of us are very skinny and some are more-naturally on the heavier side. Even our bone size and structure can vary, just as traits like our metabolic rate and length of arms and legs do. But, when it comes to improving our overall physique, it's important that you understand your variation of genetic traits, including your body type.

As a matter of interest, a keen psychologist (W.H. Sheldon, who worked in the 1940s) surmised that humans can be divided into three basic body types. And although not all individuals fall neatly into a single type, understanding these divisions can help you to build a workout that's securely optimized for your genetic type and traits. So, here are the basics of the three main body types that were given, followed by some great tips to customize workouts for each of them.

**Skinny Ectomorph Type:**

We all know people in this type and category. The ones who seem to be able to eat all they want whenever they want, without loading on any extra weight at all? Well, these people are probably ectomorphs. They are naturally slim or lean. The main downside to this type is that they have an exceptionally difficult time building up their muscle mass.

As with all types, height alone isn't a be-all and end-all factor. In fact, the types are determined by a variety of accumulations and include skeletal proportions, bone density, and metabolism as major input factors. It can be surmised (on average) though, that ectomorphs usually have narrow shoulders, lean hips, fast metabolisms, and a smaller bone structure in general terms. Their knees, wrists and ankles are usually-always smaller than the average.

## Square Endomorph Type:

Endomorphs have a thick-set bone structures and square-type torsos. This is usually accentuated by a wide waist and larger set hips. With this type, the joints are often thick, and their metabolisms are, in fact, altogether much slower.

Adding mass to their bodies is easy for this type. Their real issue is getting rid of any excess. In fact, to get lean, they must be very adherent to eating properly and getting lots of cardiovascular exercise to burn off the excess.

## Perfect Mesomorph Type:

Many of the greatest bodybuilders in history are of this type. This type has bone structures that naturally form the V-tapered look. Additionally, they are with excellent joints large enough to support increased bodybuilding mass, but still of a good size; enough to set off an appealing visual appearance. In addition, one that's proportional to (and able to) accentuate both the muscle mass and joint formations with ease. Luckily, this body type is genetically geared up to gain mass, and not add fat onto the body.

# 5

# WORKING OUT FOR YOUR SPECIFIC BODY TYPE

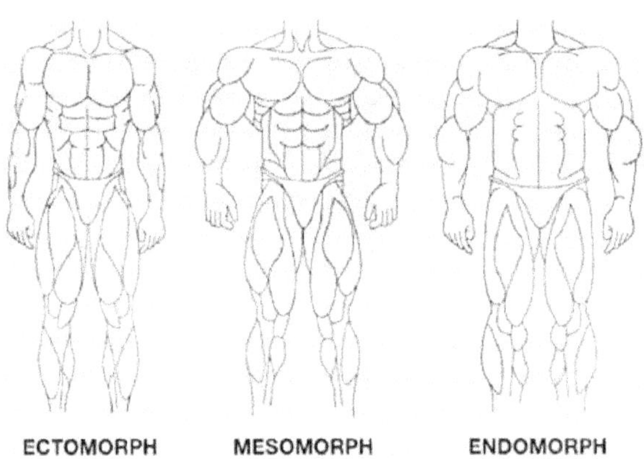



Most individuals aren't all one particular type set. You might not be totally ectomorph, endomorph or mesomorph. So, now it seems like it could get tricky. But it won't; don't worry!

It's alright, and there's no need to panic, because you're probably closer to one body type than any other. So, go with the one that fits the best. Then you can learn how to train for that one.

## Ectomorph Training

These types must be careful not to over train, and make sure they allow a maximum amount of time for both rest and recovery. Actually, ectomorphs should probably not train for more than two days in a row. The metabolism is geared so that this works out best.

In addition, the workouts should be quick and "matter-of-fact," rather than long, arduous, overbearing sessions. A time limit of one hour for any workout is the maximum required. Additionally, remaining focused on basic, compound movements and sets within the 8-10 rep requirement range, work well too. This type should not do higher reps, drop sets, super sets, or other intense paces that will strain recovery time. It's best not to add other physical activities (on top of workouts) and it's also very important that these types rest as much as possible in-between time.

Overall, to improve muscle mass, avoiding the addition of long cardio routines is crucial, because these can tear down muscle tissue. The most important thing to do for these types, is to focus the majority of the attention on preserving energy. This is so they can build, not break down, any subsequent muscle mass.

## Endomorph Training

These slower metabolism types benefit well from greater (overall) volume and frequency, when it comes to training. Additionally, doing heavy, more-focused, cardio training is advisable.

When this type focuses on lifting heavier weights, they can actually gain extra fat. If that's not an issue on an individual level, then these types can power lift with lower reps and targeted rest between sets. To target bodybuilding only, and to carry less body fat, keeping the rest periods short is a key factor. A faster pace will burn off loads more calories, and the inclusion of super sets and drop sets will too. Keeping in line with a 10-12 rep range for the upper parts of the body, and then staying at around 12-20 reps for the lower body is suggested.

For this type, it's also important to maintain an even mix of both compound and isolation movements in a balanced way. Exercises such as squats and deadlifts will really help with metabolism functioning. These will burn far more calories than exercises like leg extensions or cable cross-overs, as examples. Skipping rest days is paramount for this type, too. Actually, for days that they're not weight training or going to the gym, cardio should be the main focus point.

## Mesomorph Training

Here, these types can do any hard and consistent training. And, more than likely, they'll probably yield spectacular results no matter what they do. In fact, they can work out for longer periods and target muscle groups more frequently, blessedly - with the ability to make major gains. Actually, working harder works amazingly-well for these types.

So yes, workouts can be longer, in the 1 hour to the 90-minute range, and they should be made up of a mix of both compound and isolation movements. Repetitions can be between the (smaller) 4-6 range or as large as the 15-20 range.

These types can really make fantastic progress, they should train with a smaller volume and frequency compared to a chemically-bound enthusiast. With regard to cardio exercise, these types should do that in moderation.

# 6

# BASIC TRAINING PRINCIPLES

- Progressive Resistance
- Reps
- Training to Failure
- Sets
- Full Range of Motion
- Warming Up
- Power Training
- Resting Between Sets
- Breathing
- Stretching

When you are weight training, it is imperative to have an excellent, rounded training regime. These following training principles will show how best to benefit. Let's take a look.

## Progressive Resistance

The objective here is to build muscles in the weaker areas of your body. This is done by increasing the weights used in any particular exercise at each successive training session.

A good example being: In the first week of training, you perform barbell curls using 120 lbs. And you do ten repetitions. During the second week of training, you would increase your weights to 125 pounds. And then do another ten repetitions.

This way of exercising works on the **overload principle** where our bodies adapt to the exercise being performed. The benefits only show when the load is continually increased, and our bodies become accustomed to this new weight.

The resistance part is defined as the load which is used by the body to cause the muscles to contract.

## Reps

This is the abbreviated form of repetitions and means how many times you perform each exercise. In principle, the lighter the weight, the more repetitions you are able to do, and the heavier the weight, the fewer repetitions you will be able to do.

It might seem an obvious explanation, yet it does have a bearing on specific exercises and how they can benefit you; especially when you take a look at training intensity.

This, in simple terms, means the more reps you lift a weight for, the lower your training intensity. And likewise; the fewer reps you can do, the higher your training intensity.

All of this comes into play, as certain levels of intensity are more suited to reaching your goals than others.

To give you a good idea on how it affects your training, you can check out the following:

- 5-8 Reps per Set = Strength and Muscle Equal
- 8-10 Reps per Set = Muscle and Some Strength
- 10-12 Reps per Set = Muscle and Some Endurance
- 12-15 Reps per Set = Endurance and Some Muscle

### Training to Failure

Training to failure is the repetition of an exercise to a point where your body is unable to do one more repetition. This form of exercising helps with inducing the maximum muscle growth due to an increase of blood being pumped into that area.

If you are new to training, it has been said that training to failure can have harmful effects on your body. It is at this point, where it is advisable to begin with a rep and set regime until you have become accustomed to your regime.

It is not the physical side of the exercises that determine this advice. And, it is a fact that novices use inferior techniques while trying to train to failure, and this impedes their overall progress.

Benefits from training to failure include the boosting of strength levels, passing training plateaus, and being able to achieve the ultimate pump and maximum growth. It is used for intermediate (and up) levels of fitness, to be most beneficial.

### Sets

Generally, a set consists of a number of repetitions. Yet there are many types of sets which you can perform for a specific exercise. When you are creating a program, you have to decide how many sets you are going to perform and how many reps will be in each set.

**Straight Sets** – These are performed by beginners where the sets and the reps are the same with no change in weight.

**Compound Sets** – These consist of two exercises for the same group of muscles.

**Super Sets** – These consist of a pair of two exercises which targets two opposing muscle groups.

**Tri-Sets** – Here, three exercises are performed one after another without any break.

**Giant Sets** – This is a series of four to six exercises which are done with little rest between the movements, although there is a rest of a couple of minutes between sets.

**Drop Sets** – With this set type, you begin with heavier weights and low rep numbers and then lower the weight and perform the reps until failure.

## Full Range of Motion

A full range of motion is the act of moving as far as is possible in any given exercise. This benefits the body, especially when you wish to work a muscle to the extreme. This is because it works the whole muscle rather than just a part of it.

By doing this, the full range of motion gives: a better balance in the muscle, sustained stability in the joints, and the improvement of your movement quality.

This method of exercising is essential if you don't do a full range of motion when away from the gym. A lot of office workers sit behind a desk and have limited ranges of motion throughout the day. This leads to stiffness in the joints and then soreness, due to a lack of movement.

## Warming Up

This is one of the most important steps of any weight training program you can do. It is also done to perform one specific thing; to prevent injury.

Regular static stretching during a warm-up can rob your muscles of much-needed strength when you come to lift. It is much more beneficial to perform dynamic warm-ups. A good dynamic warm-up can consist of the following:

- 2-3 minutes of jump rope
- 20 bodyweight squats
- 10 hip extensions
- 10-20 push-ups
- 5 lunges (for each leg)
- 10 forward leg swings (for each leg)
- 10 side leg swings (for each leg)
- 50 jumping jacks

As part of your warm-up, you can use just the bars when you are aiming to work with a barbell or dumbbell, and this will get your body ready for the movements you will perform.

## Power Training

Power training focuses on reducing the overall time it will take for you to apply a specific amount of force. As your speed of movement increases, the force decreases, so, the aim is to find the correct amount of load. This then enables you to have quick movement while (at the same time) generating a sufficient amount of force.

Training for power helps to develop fast-twitch muscle fibers, along with improvements in the nervous system. This allows the body to perform rapid, explosive moments when you need a burst of power.

To develop power requires heavy weight, high sets, and a low number of reps. A good example being four or five sets of three reps - or even seven to eight sets with one or two reps.

## Resting Between Sets

This will vary depending on your goals. No matter if you wish to be stronger, more muscular, or if you wish for an increase in stamina. You can only pursue one goal at once. Focus on your goal to decide.

## Strength Training

If you are training for strength, then three to five minutes rest between sets is recommended. This allows the body to re-charge the ATP-PC system. This is the ability of the oxidative system to use fats, carbohydrates and protein as fuel. This then allows you to lift more weight and you can get stronger in a shorter period of time.

## Hypertrophic Training

If you wish to get bigger quicker, you will rest for one to two minutes between sets. These shorter rest periods create an increase in blood flow and lactate production to your targeted muscles.

## Stamina (Endurance) Training

If you are training for stamina, you would only rest for forty-five seconds to two minutes, between sets. This helps the muscles to be resilient against fatigue as your body is able to clear lactic acid more efficiently.

**Breathing:**

It might sound simple enough, yet the idea of breathing isn't just about how you inhale and exhale during exercising. When you breathe properly, it can aid in increasing abdominal power to help improve recovery time between your exercise sets.

The correct way to breathe is inhaling while you are performing the eccentric part of the exercise, and then exhaling during the concentric part of the exercise.

Stability is improved when you breathe appropriately, because it is what you would know as "bracing." This extra stability while bracing the abdominal muscles helps to burn more calories and move more weigh

Breathing is also essential for relaxing and recovering. If you are breathing hard, you'll notice you are chest breathing. If you breathe from the abdominals rather than the chest, you can take much deeper breaths which will aid in recovery.

**Stretching:**

Stretching is not just important in your warm-ups, it can also help to increase strength, speed and muscle growth. It can also aid in a quicker recovery time.

To aid in muscle growth by stretching, you should perform these stretches during training (rather than before or after). When performing stretches during training, they should be done on the muscles you have just worked, and for periods of not less than sixty seconds.

With intense stretching, you should be at the point of where it begins to hurt, and as a guide, your body will quickly let you know when you have gone too far. When you reach this hurting point, and have held it for sixty seconds, be careful to release your muscles very gradually. This prevents injury.

Hypertrophy (increased skeletal muscle) can be increased with the use of exercise stretching mostly because it releases growth factors in the muscles. And these being; hepatocyte growth factor, myogenin, and IGF-1. It might be annoying or time consuming at the time, yet it does work wonders.

# ISOMETRICS: THE SECRET KEY TO SUPER STRENGTH

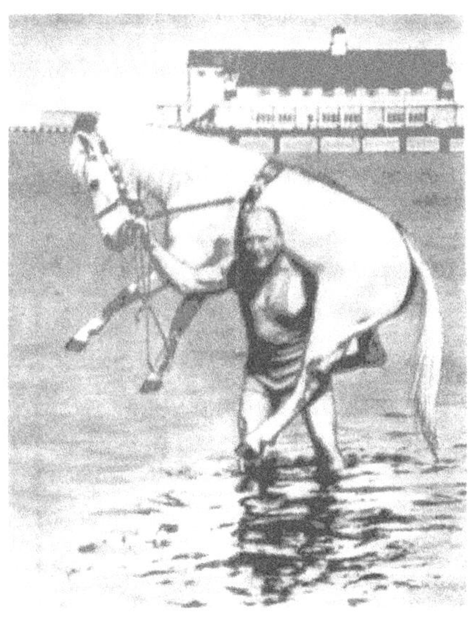

IF THERE WERE ANY REAL SECRETS IN THE WORLD OF SUPER strength, this is definitely the be-all and end-all. When done properly, using isometrics gets you past any plateau which can be the difference between ongoing success or failure. A highly underestimated tool, it's no wonder it is one of the most negated forms of strength training. But… those that know this powerful secret, hold the wisdom to unlock true, superhuman potential, or powers.

Remaining focused is the most important aspect of any exercise system. And whether it's muscle control, lifting weights, rep training, or even going for extended periods of time in one exercise form, the difference remains the same. Yes, isometrics really takes on an exceptionally new level of focus, and a much-needed, perfected concentration level that is accurate and on point. It doesn't matter if you hold a position for 12 seconds or 12 hours, the focus is still required. It takes monumental focus and concentration, and not just within the physical body, but also internally as a focal point of belief. The real secret with isometrics is not how long you can hold any posture, position or contraction… the real power is in how much internal power you can attain and hold for the period of integration. This *IS* the secret.

One of the world's (quite possibly the greatest) renowned wrestlers, The Great Gama, was a testament to the sport as an incredible athlete. In fact, Gama was well-known for his unbelievably-brutal workout training, ranging from swimming right through to wrestling. He even did some exercises for hours on end. Additionally, the massive amount of repetitions he achieved for both push-ups and squats were phenomenal. On a global scale, he was famous for never losing a match in his entire career, which was 5000 matches in total. An unbelievable human being.

Gama was fierce with both his renowned takedown and throwing techniques, and he could toss his opponents without any real effort, or so it seemed. Part of his training entailed tying a belt or a strap around a tree. He would then try with every ounce of his strength and internal focus to take down that tree. Gama also incorporated other forms of isometrics too, and his opponents were not really excited about facing him in the wrestling ring, for understandable reasons. He was fierce and all-powerful. We will touch on him some more, soon, a little later in the title.

It's important to understand that the major practice of isometrics is best done by working them into your own training regimen, or just doing them as they were intended. This is because, great practice methods that (historically) work, have already been researched and trialed well, so we know that they can create the success we seek. If you can stay open-minded, you'll find yourself in a wonderful new world of strength training. One that's more successful, healthier, and much more efficient to your body's needs, as opposed to the weight machines, cardio machines, and the vast array of dumbbells you see being utilized these days. So yes, we can find a unique methodology of real strength training and great, purposeful ability from some of the greats. The ones who did it for real, historically. We'll take a look at them soon, so stay tuned for that.

Prior to weight lifting equipment and the ushering in of up-to-date gyms, individuals who sought to increase size and strength used to push against stationary objects. A straightforward way to see this is by locking your hands together and pushing back against yourself with as much force as possible.

To simplify the fact, muscles only contract in specific ways. One of the most obvious ways is when contracting and shortening the muscle lengths when doing bicep curls. The technical term for this is concentric contraction, and this is where muscles tense while they contract (shorten in length).

Muscles are also able to tense while they lower loads (or resist against them). This would occur when dropping the arm back to the starting position in a bicep curl. This contraction type is termed eccentric, and this arises as the muscle becomes tense as it lengthens.

Another muscle contraction is known as an isometric contraction which occurs when the muscles tense without any change in their length. Prime examples are when body-building posing or when pushing against objects which are immovable, such as walls. Isometric training possesses the main benefits where the body can activate almost all of the available motor units to some degree; this is typically, extremely hard to accomplish.

Way back during the 1950s, scientists Hettinger and Muller established a single daily effort of around two-thirds of a person's possible maximum. When exerted for a period of only six seconds at a time, and performed over a ten week period, strength increased by around 5% each week.

Clark and associates established that static strength carried on increasing, even after a five-week regimen of isometric exercises had concluded. Additional benefits of isometric training are purely the total time spent performing any given exercise. When considering exercises like bench presses, it might take one or two seconds to perform the action for each joint angle. Each muscle only needs training for reduced periods of time.

On the contrary, exercises which mimic bench presses, such as a press against pins at the locking position of a lift, well, these might need to be performed for more than a few seconds. What this means is, if you find you have problems at specific joint angles during your lift, you can use targeted isometrics which helps to alleviate your problems, right then and there.

Typically, as soon as we raise weights, our muscles absorb type-2 fiber. It is once we start approaching our maximum effort of 100% that the body forces itself to engage its fast-twitch muscle fibers. If this were not to happen, these would then become neglected. When training in this nature, we see results in increased strength as micro-tears are created in the most powerful cells in the muscles, and which increase as they heal. Amazing!

To fully use 100% effort, we have only two techniques in which we can use. Either we can lift 100% of our one rep maximum capacity, or we can lift around 85% of maximum capacity, but with increased speed and explosiveness. This varies to our regular exercises, with the lifting of heavy weights and employing bursts of explosive speed. This requires the body to generate additional force. It is this occurrence that helps our muscle strength increase.

Holding weights in position until we feel a complete fatigue is an alternative way oof movement. And this utilizes the fast-twitch muscle fibers of the body, as it does when you push or pull against an object which you are unable to move. When merely pushing or pulling against an object which you are unable to move, ultimately your body starts adapting to be in the condition to move this object over time. Additionally, this also goes a long way to create stronger "neural drives" between the brain and muscles. And as it happens, when you command your body to use all of its muscle, you then also increase the ability to engage muscle fiber at will. Feedback is also forthright as you start feeling that your muscles are working. As fast-twitch muscle fibers are the most significant type, these are the best to increase hypertrophy and show a visible increase in muscle size.

## How Strong Can We Really Get?

At the beginning of the 20th century, the world started to see the introduction of a previously unseen kind of public hero: professional strongmen. These strongmen arose from physical culture movements which were built during the 1800s as a response to what we now know as the Industrial Revolution.

With the explosion of office working, there was an increasing concern in what way this new deskbound lifestyle was affecting overall health — and "manliness," for the men of the nation.

Strongmen became symbols of preserved virility, and living proof the male citizens still possessed grit, power, and the strength of their ancestors, with the potential for performing macho, or masculine activities. If men were no longer able to tame the wild frontier, and face the challenges of nature, they, in turn, could become masters of themselves, and then pit their resoluteness against the weights and feats of the strength of a gymnasium. And so, strongmen arrived from all corners of the world, and diverse cultural backgrounds, too. Some materialized from the ranks of professional and amateur athletes. They were previously boxers, wrestlers, or participants in the Olympics (and the lesser-known Highland games).

Some previously served as physical training instructors in the military forces, while others had merely been in laborious jobs like those of blacksmiths or factory laborer positions. Here, they saw the chance to make a decent living by using their brawn in a less tedious and grueling way. Strongmen found no shortage of where to ply their trade. Even displaying feats of strength and prowess in floor show acts, which were performed in music halls and the many dime-store museums. The lifting of these heavy weights as an end, was in fact, an unusual-enough concept, and so it grabbed the attention of, and captivated the public audiences. They were willing to pay to watch powerfully-built men hoist dumbbells, barbells, and other peculiarly-formed objects.

Strongmen broadened their acts while incorporating stunts. The barehanded breaking of chains, tearing decks of cards in half, and bending iron bars and horseshoes. This was the leadup to pulling large items by only their teeth, and also engrossing the crowds with mock gladiatorial tournaments.

Many deceptions were performed in these shows. With entertainers using trickery and deception to pull off their perceptible deeds of strength. Nonetheless, there were genuine strength participants on the show circuits, who did insist that it was to be manpower alone when performing their lifts and stunts.

These strongmen turned out to be, not only the promoters of engaging sideshows, but they also aided to evolve an awareness of physical cultures and overall fitness to a broader public audience. Naturally, regular men wanted to know how they too could build similar physiques, especially after seeing these strongmen perform.

A number of these strongmen went on to create numerous books and mail-order courses. These courses laid out the suggested strength-building programs. They remained immensely available in the first half of the 20th century. Such was the impact; they helped to launch a fitness (awareness) culture which still remains as a part of our history, even today.

Some of the acts that strongmen performed involved many classic lifts and exercises. A number of these are still recognized today (although much of what is considered good form has been improved over time), like the squat, jerk and clean, and more. Some other exercises were truly unique and have now mostly-been forgotten since the zenith of these old-time strongmen.

If the effects of isometric training still don't have you convinced, then ponder over the thought for a moment, it is the foundation of some of the world's strongest people ever born. They realized their abilities and capabilities by utilizing isometrics.

How strong can we really become? Well, when talking about some of the legendary strongmen feats, you can quickly get the idea of how authentically-amazing our bodies are and what they really can achieve.

## A Great Hero of Our Time

## Alexander Zass – The Iron Samson

## 1888 - 1962

Alexander Zass was born in Vilna, Poland. However, he spent his younger years living in Russia. Like countless other strongmen of his period, Zass was driven to increase his strength after attending a circus and seeing the exploits performed by the circus strongman there.

Zass began with the bending of green branches, climbing trees and running with his home-made dumbbells and barbells. It was later that he trained beneath some of the most-famous, professional, Russian strongmen.

Zass developed incredible strength which allowed him to transport a horse on his shoulders. His most momentous talents were the bending of steel bars and the breaking of chains, which became the centerpiece of his exhibitions.

**Interesting Fact:** In 1914, while he served in the Russian army at some stage in the First World War, Zass became wounded and was taken prisoner by Austrian forces. As a prisoner of war, he persistently developed his strength by using isometrics. He did this by pulling on the bars and chains. Zass ultimately escaped from his prison and never returned to his homeland.

Out of all the strongmen, he is without a doubt, my favorite. There are a few old black and white videos of him performing some of his crazy feats.

*"I aimed first, to develop the underlying connective tissues rather than the superficial muscles. I developed tendon strength. The tendons are the cord-like media between the bones and the muscles. A large bicep is no more criterion of strength than a swollen abdomen is of digestion. It is the pulling tendon of the biceps that counts. Moreover, so on throughout the whole body, this method was employed. Some men with thin legs are stronger than some with thick legs. Why? Because strength lies in the tendons; they are the powerful fibrous attachments of the muscles to the bones. They are, in short, the master key to the strength which overcomes great resistance. Without tendons, one would possess no control over the body. There would be no rigidity, no steadiness of physical movement. They, and their development, are the secret of my strength. I am tendon-strong. Muscles alone won't hold horses back. Tendons will; and do. But they must be cultivated. Oh, yes. They must be developed. There is a way of increasing their strength, and that way, I claim in all modesty, I have perfected. Real, sound, and efficient is my method."* - Alexander Zass

## 7 Reasons You Need Radical Hand Strength

I made a fundamental observation over the years regarding the bulk of men who work out. They disregard the importance of training with the hands. Keeping this in mind, I thought I'd go through and swiftly list a few reasons you should build your own incredible hand strength.

1 – No longer do you have to get your mom, your girlfriend or other

female relatives to open stubborn jars for you! This should be self-explanatory. Nevertheless, there is a broader argument behind it. We'll explore in more detail later. I added this one for fun!

2 – Your hands lead the body. From the messages the nervous system sends your body, it actually thinks your hands are enormous. They contain twice the number of nerve endings compared to other parts of the body. When you exercise and train your hands to be strong, you are, in fact, helping to condition your nerves. This nerve force is a fundamental component of health and strength, and it was definitely a massive factor for the old-time strongmen of yesteryear.

3 – The hands help to make more of your physical power useable. You will have the ability to lift heavier weight using your back, legs, and shoulders too. This applies to the more significant muscle groups of the body. Unfortunately, what stops many people in the real world, is the lack of strength in their hands. If you can generate 500 lbs. of force with your legs and back, but your hands can only accommodate 300 lbs., then you inefficiently limit yourself in the real world, which is unfortunate, but true.

4 – Hand's help to stimulate the entire body. Again, we traverse back to the nerves. Most movements we perform in the old-time strongman tradition show us that hand training helps to stimulate the body. If you aspire to increase health, more muscle, more strength, then it's necessary. It's time to kick your body into gear from a nerve and hormonal point of view. The hands have to be trained hard with immense exercises that give the whole body a workout.

5 – Many hand exercises aid in building serious muscle. Take a look at two of the top students of the old-time arts - Mike "The Machine" and Bruce and Pat "The Human Vise" Povilaitis – Both possess enormous muscular development. Now, do they do other forms of training? They do, absolutely, yes. However, they also perform lots of bending, and this is BIG bending! When this is implemented well, this bending works several muscles inside, and these small muscles

you are unable to see. If you wish to build some serious muscle and make sure it's a muscle that's fully functional, make sure to work your hands with strongman training.

6 – Your hand strength is able to save lives! It is quite sad to know that there are a lot of people who cannot pull themselves over a wall. This could be out of the way of a flood, an emergency situation that could require a quick exit from an area, or any other life-threatening situation. A large part of the reason is due to great hand strength, and if hands are too weak, then they will (subsequently) let an individual down. Most modern society activities do not need exceptional hand strength. Nevertheless, that should not stop you possessing what you ought to have. Tremendous hand strength, and the natural ability to use those hands in ways that are practical is paramount. And in ways that can literally save people's lives.

7 – For self-defense. A vast number of people think the modern world is safer than it actually is. Let's be truthful – there are places around the world, even in America, that are nowhere close to being safe. The stronger you can make your hands, the better chance you have to defend yourself and that of a partner or family member.

You need strong hands! By training with the strongman feats in the same way I do, this is one of the best ways for building hand strength. It is a fact, and it's not only a great way of increasing hand strength, but you will also find you can have a lot of fun in the process. At the end of it, you will have the great sense of accomplishment, too.

If you're interested in isometrics and the famous strongman of old, checkout my title "Super Strength," it contains bucket loads of information and over 20 old strongman isometric exercises all for Free! Click here!

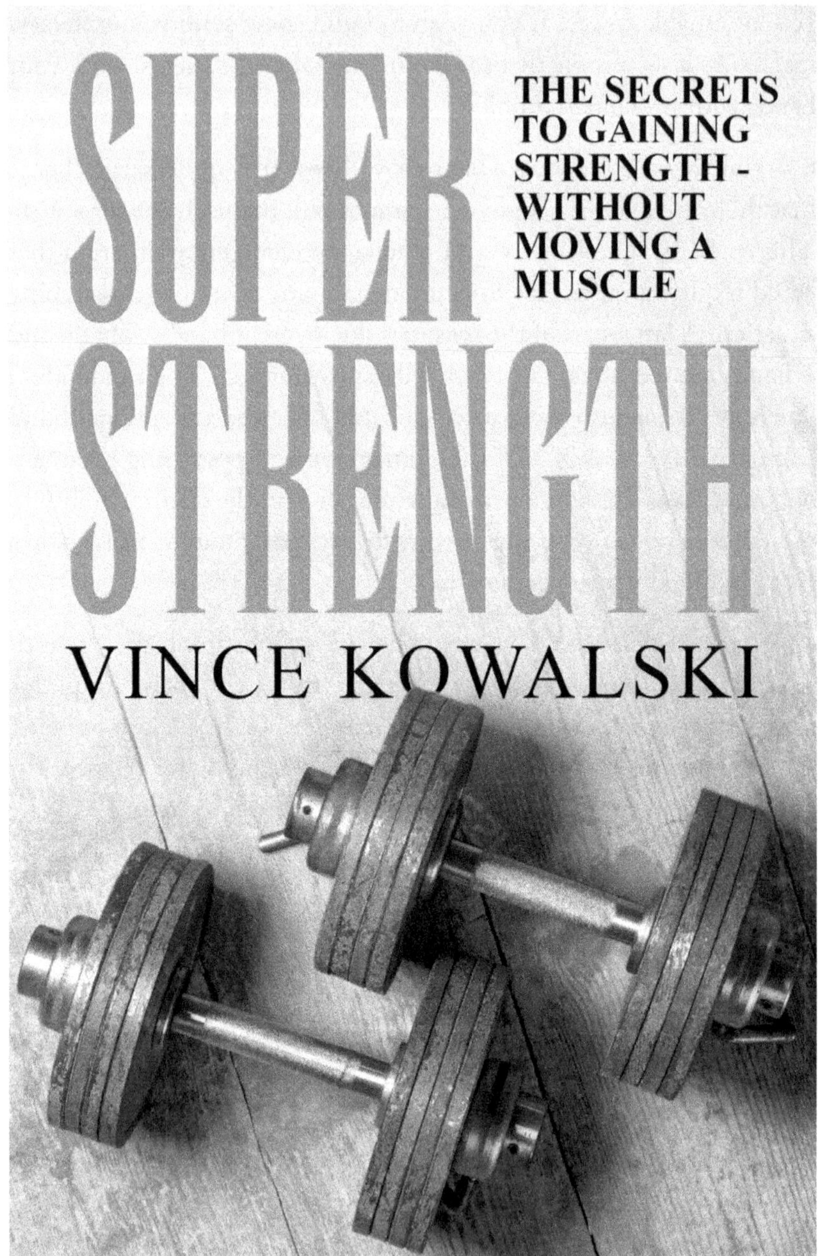
SUPER
STRENGTH
THE SECRETS
TO GAINING
STRENGTH -
WITHOUT
MOVING A
MUSCLE
VINCE KOWALSKI

# HOW THE DIET INFLUENCES YOUR TRAINING

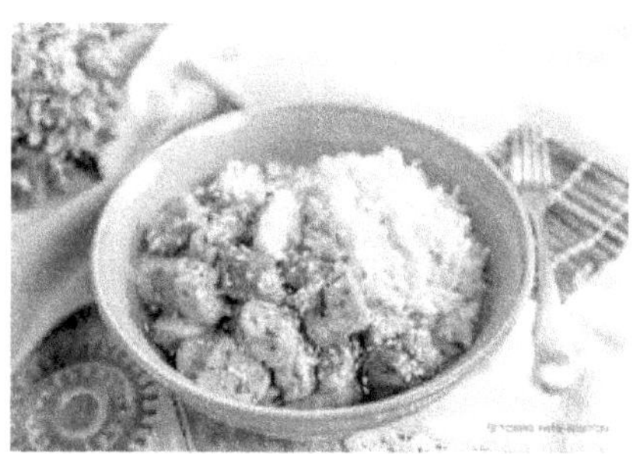

TRAINING PROMOTES MUSCLE GROWTH. BUT FOR THIS TRAINING to work well, your body needs a decent and efficient amount of energy, and enough of the right type of foods to get the full benefit from your exercise program/s. Providing the source of great energy is the role nutrition plays in anabolic functioning.

Nutrition can help you to stay lean, mean, and become muscular. In fact, understanding how much and what kinds of food to eat for the best possible result, is paramount. By definition, learning the basic nutrients available and determining how much of each one you need, is vital to the cause.

Great nutrition also is also concerned utilizing the right protein, excellent vitamins, vital minerals, and other supplements too. Knowing how not only helps you get larger and stronger, but it also keeps you heathier. This is because great nutrition supports your immune system and aids long-term health.

Additionally, the benefits of good nutrition also include: enhancing your recovery time from big workouts, giving you awesome skin, producing excellent functioning of the liver, and allowing other internal organs to thrive well.

Now we can understand how important the basic principles of nutrition are. They actually aid the good principles of any training regime. Yes, nutrition is absolutely essential to accentuating and growing a strong, healthy, amazing-looking body. And should be given the same importance as your workouts. Did you know that exercise creates a demand for nutrients? And the kinds of nutrients you provide is a major, detrimental factor in producing the kind of results you want. Especially long-term.

The main purpose of nutrition in bodybuilding is to help you gain muscle and also lose fat. Many popular diets are concerned with losing overall body weight, but many of them result in losing way too much muscle tissue, as well as stored body fat. Some individuals half-starve themselves in an attempt to achieve maximum muscularity, but this won't work. Please don't do this. Your body cannot thrive if it is starved. Let's go over some of the basics, now.

The All-Important Basics

The 4 basic nutrients known as macronutrients are:

1. **Protein**

Protein is composed of different types of amino acids, and they provide the building blocks for muscle tissue. Protein makes up a component for all organs, and it's also importantly involved in the structures of the skin, the bones, the tendons, additionally, being involved in many bodily functions (because all enzymes are proteins).

1. **Carbohydrates**

Carbohydrates give us much-needed fuel for energy. Carbohydrates are composed of a large variety of less-complex or more-complex sugar and starch molecules.

1. **Fats (or oils)**

Fats (or oils) are the nutrients that hold the most densely-packed energy stores.

1. **Water**

Water is also a vital nutrient. It actually constitutes a whopping 72% of muscle in the body.

The purpose of a great diet in bodybuilding is to help you to gain muscle and also lose fat. Many fad diets are concerned with losing overall body weight, but many of them result in losing a substantial amount of muscle tissue, along with stored body fat. Some individuals half-starve themselves in an attempt to achieve maximum muscular builds. Don't do this, it's unnecessary and very, very dangerous for your health.

Diet with Regard to Body Types: Ectomorphs:

When it comes to eating for controlling body composition, the first type are ectomorphs (an individual with a lean and delicate build). Ectomorphs have a fast metabolism. They tend to be able to turn food into energy easily and quickly. These types of individuals need to eat high protein and to increase overall caloric intake as well. Needing more calories, they'll often benefit from having excess fat in their diets, when compared to the other two body types.

## Mesomorphs:

Mesomorphs (are muscular, naturally and well-built with a high metabolism and very responsive muscle cells). These bodies easily turn food into muscle. They distinctly require high protein for muscle maintenance and development. These types can consume a relatively normal number of calories, because they are able to burn off fat effectively.

## Endomorphs:

Endomorphs (slower metabolisms and a greater number of fat cells). Additionally, these types of individuals also have a strong inclination to turn ingested food into body fat that gets stored. They must consume enough protein, and they need to keep their calorie intake to a minimum so as not to store more fat. It's important that they make sure that only 20% of calories comes from a fat source. Approximately 20% of endomorphs have a lower than average thyroid output, and this adds to the problem. This type needs to work harder at keeping lean and slim, but they tend to build up their muscle relatively effectively, especially when compared to the ectomorph type. Additionally, they can eventually lose more excess body fat through utilizing a great diet, and a well-structured exercise program.

Awesome Shakes for Bodybuilding

Any seasoned fitness veteran will tell you, that when it comes to receiving the best calories, nothing is more viable than a high-quality, whole-food meal. If you aim to get bigger, it is a well-known fact that you need to eat big! However, the full benefits that a protein-packed shake can deliver, are second-to-none. They are full of high-quality protein and packed with nutrients and healthy calories. They are also absorbed by the body quicker than eating a full, sit-down meal. When used correctly, one or two of these shakes throughout the day will help you to quickly achieve your desired goals.

## Shake the Vanilla & Coffee

Forget the coffee shop coffee which is packed full of sugar. Try this much-healthier alternative.

### Ingredients

- 1 1/2 cups of low-fat milk
- 2 scoops of vanilla protein powder
- 1/2 a cup low-fat ice cream, coffee flavored

### Directions

Add all ingredients to a blender and mix until well combined. Pour and enjoy.

## Soy Almond Shake

Plant protein can be used instead of Greek yogurt for a vegan alternative.

### Ingredients

- 1 scoop of whey protein powder – plain or vanilla
- 1 cup of light soy milk
- 1 tablespoon of sliced almonds
- 1 teaspoon of sugar-free maple syrup (or honey)
- 3 drops of vanilla extract
- 1 handful of ice cubes
- 1 tablespoon of low-fat Greek yogurt (omit for vegan)

**Directions**

Add all to a blender and mix until well combined. Pour and enjoy.


Early Bird Shake

Boost your breakfast and your immune system with vitamin C. Do this with the brightness of fresh oranges.

**Ingredients**

- 3 large oranges, for juice (not canned or bottled)
- sweetener, to taste (optional- honey)
- 1 scoop of whey protein powder – plain or vanilla

**Directions**

Add all to a blender and mix until well combined. Pour and enjoy.


Sweet & Nutty Oatmeal Shake

Forget cooking oatmeal, this is one for the road. Great for on-the-go!

**Ingredients**

- 1 cup of dry oatmeal
- 2 scoops of whey protein powder – plain or vanilla
- 1/2 teaspoon of cinnamon
- 1/8 cup of sugar-free maple syrup (honey, optional)
- 1 tablespoon of chopped almonds
- 1 1/2 cups of low-fat milk (can use water)
- **Directions**

Add all to a blender and mix until well combined. Pour and enjoy.

## High-Protein Snacks: Edamame

Packed full of protein and have lots of complex carbs and fat to give you a long-lasting energy boost. Soybeans are also chock-full of folate, vitamin K, magnesium, and iron.

## Pumpkin Seeds

Pumpkin seeds contain 7 grams of protein for each serving, which is a great consideration when you look at their size. They don't contain any sugars and are a great addition to salads, oatmeal, yogurts, or with cottage cheese.

## Pouched Fish

With these, you don't need to drain them or carry a can opener. All you need is your fork, and your snack is ready. The proteins will fill you for much longer when they are mixed with fats or fiber. Try adding some guacamole into the pouch as it contains both.

## Hard-Boiled Eggs

Eggs are well known to be rich in BCAAs which can help to build muscle.

It is easy to boil a few in one go and keep them by your side at work. Also, there's no need for the trip to the vending machine. Omega-3 enriched, these are the best source of goodness for the brain.

## Delicious Soups

Studies repeatedly show when diners consume low-calorie, vegetable-based soups before their main meal, they can, on average, consume up to 20% fewer calories per meal. The reason is quite simple. The bulkiness of the soup will help to fill us up, so we end up eating considerably less. This is also beneficial nutritionally, because all of the nutrients found in the vegetables also include vitamins such as vitamins B, C, K, and dietary fiber. Also, a full range of minerals can be found, which helps in regulating the digestive tract. This also ensures we acquire the much-needed vital nutrients we require each day for great health and functioning, on a cellular, metabolic level.

Eating soups can also have an extra benefit when you look at them from a weight and fluid retention standpoint. Soups that have the main base of leeks, onions, and celery, come loaded with the mineral called potassium.

Potassium aids in binding excess sodium (salt), and it helps the body to rid it of excess fluid. A vast number of us carry retained fluid, and on a regular basis we may feel bloated, which is (unfortunately) thanks to a diet which is high in salt and coupled with a lack of activity. This is especially true if we've followed a western-inspired one.

While meals can be bulked up with low-calorie vegetable soups, eating them on a regular basis is a fantastic way to load up on nutrition overall, especially for anyone wanting to shed a few kilos, speedily. And the replacement of the evening meal with vegetable-based soups is definitely a safe and healthy way of achieving this.

The low energy content of soups helps in keeping your overall total of calorie content low. As an aside, the bulk helps prevent you from feeling overly hungry and feeling deprived. This is what happens if you were eating limited amounts, like you would have to do on a conventional diet, or (alternatively) if you were using one of the many meal replacement shakes which are available.

Oven Roasted Tomato Soup: Ingredients

- 10 large tomatoes - cut into quarters
- 1 tablespoon of virgin olive oil
- 1/2 a teaspoon of kosher salt
- 1/4 teaspoon of ground black pepper
- 1/4 of a cup of balsamic vinegar
- 2 cups of vegetable broth - low-sodium
- 1/2 cup of skimmed milk
- 2 tablespoons of honey
- 1/4 cup of fresh basil, roughly chopped
- parmesan cheese - grated for sprinkling

## Directions

- Preheat the oven to 400 F. and line a baking sheet with foil. Spread the tomatoes in an even, single layer.
- Drizzle with olive oil and the balsamic vinegar. Sprinkle with salt and pepper.
- Roast for about 30 to 35 minutes, or until the tomatoes start charring a little on the edges.
- Once cooked, add the tomatoes to a blender in small batches, and then blend until smooth.
- Add water to the tomatoes if the mixture becomes too thick to blend.
- Pour the blended tomatoes into a large Dutch oven.
- On low-medium heat, add the vegetable stock, skimmed milk and the honey.
- Mix and then add the blended tomatoes to the pan.

- Stir while bringing the mixture to a simmer. Cover and simmer for another 10 minutes.
- Divide into serving bowls and sprinkle basil to garnish.
- Sprinkle grated parmesan cheese, if desired.

Slow Cooked Minestrone Soup: Ingredients

- 6 cups of vegetable broth - low-sodium
- 1 (15 ounce) can of crushed tomatoes - low-sodium
- 1 (15 ounce) can of diced tomatoes - low-sodium
- 1 (15 ounce) can of kidney beans - rinsed and drained
- 1 medium onion - diced
- 1 cup of celery - diced small
- 1 cup of carrot - diced small
- 1 cup of fresh green beans - cut into ½-inch slices
- 6 cloves of garlic - minced
- 2 teaspoons of dried oregano
- 1 teaspoon of dried basil
- 1 teaspoon of dried thyme
- 1/2 teaspoon of kosher salt
- 1/2 cup of whole-wheat elbow pasta
- 1 small zucchini, cut into cubes
- 3 cups of kale, washed and roughly chopped
- 1/2 a cup of parmesan cheese - grated
- 2 tablespoons of fresh basil, roughly chopped for garnish

## Directions

- Add all the ingredients to a slow cooker, except the pasta, zucchini, kale, parmesan, and fresh basil.
- Cook for 6 hours on low, or 4 hours on high.
- Once cooked, add the elbow pasta, the zucchini cubes, and

the kale. Cook for one additional hour on high until the pasta is tender.
- Divide into serving bowls and sprinkle with grated parmesan.
- Top with fresh basil.

## Slow-Cooked Lentil Soup: Ingredients

- 1 cup of green lentils - rinsed and drained
- 1/2 cup of red onion - chopped small
- 5 cups of vegetable broth - low-sodium
- 1/2 cup of celery - cut small
- 1/2 cup carrot - peeled and diced small
- 1 small sweet potato - peeled and diced small
- 4 cloves of garlic - minced
- 1/2 teaspoon of ground cumin
- 1/2 a lemon for zest
- 2 teaspoons of lemon juice - 1/2 a lemon
- 2 tablespoons of dried oregano
- 2 tablespoons of tomato paste
- 3 cups of fresh baby spinach - washed and drained

## Directions

- Add all the ingredients into a slow cooker, apart from the tomato paste and the baby spinach.
- Cook for 6 hours on low, or 4 hours on high.
- Once the lentils are tender, add the tomato paste, the spinach, and stir. Re-cover and cook for a further 20 minutes on high, or until the spinach has wilted.
- Divide between serving bowls and serve.

## Cream of Broccoli Soup: Ingredients

- 1 large head of broccoli - broken into florets
- 3 cups of vegetable broth - low-sodium
- 1/4 teaspoon of kosher salt
- 1/2 teaspoon of black pepper - cracked
- 1 cup of canned coconut milk

## Directions

- Steam broccoli for ten minutes, or until tender. Chop steamed florets (1/2 cup) and set aside.
- Add to a blender the first 4 ingredients (in the given order). Save the 1/2 cup of chopped florets for later. Blend until you have a creamy consistency.
- Pour the soup into a medium Dutch oven and add the remaining 1/2 a cup of chopped broccoli. Add the coconut milk, and heat over a medium heat until it's warmed through.
- Whole-grain croutons can be used for garnish if desired.

## Protein Pancakes, Crepes & Inspirations

Inspirational desserts are one of those things you can eat at any time of the day. They really aren't restricted to after dinner, either, so you can whip them up and get stuck in for some protein-packed, purposeful munching.

## Banana Fluff Pancakes: Ingredients

- 2 scoops of protein powder - vanilla flavor
- 2 large eggs - free-range

- 1 large banana - very ripe
- 1/8 of a teaspoon of cinnamon
- 1/4 of a teaspoon of baking powder
- 1/4 of a teaspoon of kosher salt
- coconut oil - for cooking

## Directions

- In a medium mixing bowl, add the egg whites and beat until soft peaks form. Around 2 minutes should suffice.
- In a second mixing bowl, add the remaining ingredients to the egg yolks and beat until smooth.
- Fold 1/3 of the egg whites into the banana and egg yolk mixture, until combined. Repeat (bit by bit) until all egg whites have been incorporated well.
- Heat a skillet over medium-high heat, add coconut oil, and then spoon out about 2 tablespoons of batter.
- Cook for 45 seconds or until the edges brown, then flip the pancake and cook for about 30-45 seconds on the second side.

X3 Almond Flour Pancake: Ingredients:

- 1 1/2 cups of blanched almond flour
- 3 large eggs - free-range
- 1 medium banana - ripe
- 1 teaspoon of baking powder
- coconut oil - for cooking
- berries and/or almond butter for topping (optional)

## Directions:

- Add all the ingredients into a blender and blend until a thick, smooth batter forms.
- Heat a skillet over medium-high heat, add coconut oil, and then spoon out about 2 tablespoons of batter.
- Cook for around 2 minutes or until the edges brown, then flip the pancake and cook the second side until browned and cooked right through.

Spinach Protein Waffles: Ingredients

- 1 large egg - free-range
- 1/3 of a cup of Greek yogurt - plain and non-fat
- 1 handful of spinach - washed and dried
- 1/3 of a cup of rolled oats
- 1/2 a packet of powdered sweetener
- coconut oil - for cooking

**Directions**

- Add all the ingredients into a blender, and blend until a thick, smooth batter forms.
- Plug in and heat up a waffle iron.
- Pour all the batter into the heated waffle iron and close.
- Cook for around 5 minutes, or until no longer steaming. Waffle should be lightly golden brown.

Peanut Butter 3-Ingredient Pancakes: Ingredients

- 1 medium banana - ripe
- 2 large eggs - free-range
- 2 tablespoons of peanut flour
- coconut oil - for cooking

## Sauce

- 1 tablespoon of peanut flour - for the sauce
- 1 1/2 tablespoons of almond milk - for the sauce

## Directions

- Add the first 3 ingredients into a blender and blend until a thick, smooth batter forms.
- Heat a skillet over medium-high heat, add coconut oil, and then spoon out about 2 tablespoons of batter.
- Cook for around 2 minutes or until the edges brown, then flip the pancake and cook the second side until browned and cooked right through.
- Add the peanut flour with the 1 1/2 tablespoons of almond milk and mix to a thick consistency. Pour over cooked pancakes.

That's all of the amazing recipes... I hope you absolutely love them all. They are geared up for their stimulation constituents, and also jam-packed full of flavor! Enjoy!

If you interested in more high protein meals and some more guidance in regard to nutrition, check out my book – Anabolic Kitchen, it has over 140 high protein, easy to make and delicious meals and it absolutely free! Click here for your copy.

# VINCE KOWALSKI

# ANABOLIC KITCHEN

## 140 RECIPES FOR STAYING LEAN, BUILDING MUSCLE AND STAYING HEALTHY FOR MEN AND WOMEN

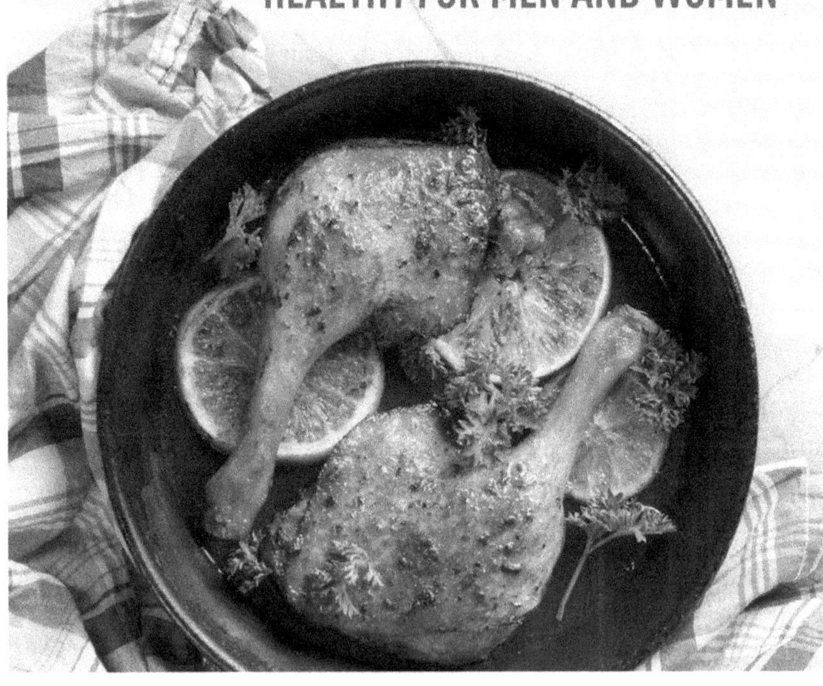

# 6-PACK ABS AND THE SCIENCE BEHIND THEM

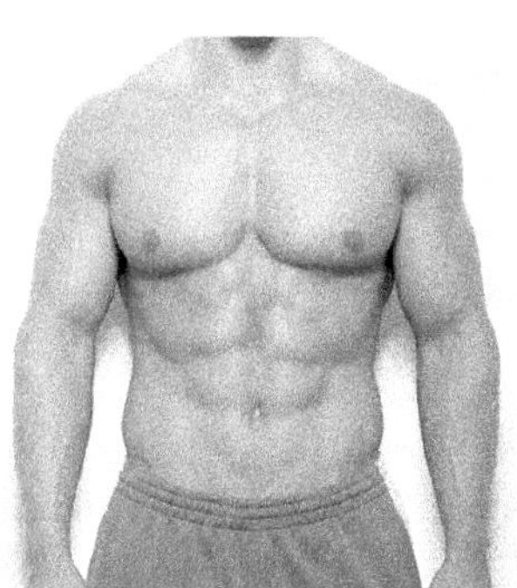

WHILE I HAVE SPOKEN IN THE PREVIOUS CHAPTER ABOUT THE importance of nutrition it's only natural that the next chapter we speak about abs and ripped six packs. The phrase, "Abs are made in the kitchen!" actually holds a lot of truth, and we've all heard it, but not everyone believes it.

Before you can get that shredded 6-pack, you first need to understand how you can achieve it from a scientific viewpoint. First up, let's understand that everyone has some form of a 6-pack. Sure, it might be hidden or shaped differently, but the amount of abdominal definition and the quality of it is reliant on a few, simple, key variables:

## Body Fat Levels

This is the overall amount of body fat your body has. For many people, this figure is too high, and you'll never be able to reveal your 6-pack unless this is lessened. You can have the world's best (hardest) abs, but if your body fat content is too high, you'll never see them (nor will anyone else).

## Abdominal Muscle Mass

Once you have become lean enough, you can do additional ab work, and the increased ab muscle mass will lead to an improvement in ab definition and thickness.

## Genetics and Abdominal Structure

Some individuals tend to store less body fat around their midriff and might seem to have been handed some excellent ab genetics, giving them a very-worthy cover model, or 6-pack look. But not to worry, even if that doesn't sound like you, my system works for all body types.

## Stubborn Areas and Body Fat Storage

Many people store surplus fat around their stomach area. This, in turn, requires them to diet a little harder and to reduce that stubborn fat around the belly, (midriff or core).

For a high number of people, the primary focus should be shedding (or stripping back) body fat. This is more crucial around the belly. Some have sufficient ab muscles (core) to give them a head-turning 6-

pack, already. All they have to do is become lean enough for it to show.

There are many lean athletes and members of the general public who never train their abs, and despite this, we can still see they have great 6-pack abs, especially when they are lean enough for it to be noticeable.

In this title, we'll learn that our primary concern ought to be an overall fat loss, and more specifically, fat loss in the belly region. Once you become leaner and can start seeing your 6-pack, then you can add some ab-specific work to help increase your abdominal density and thickness.

Body Fat Level; How Much Is Required?: Men:

With a body fat percentage below 14%, men can start showing their 6-pack form. Yet, under 10% body fat gives a broader, cover model look, allowing for a more-defined 6-pack, while revealing the lower abs, also.

**Women:**

Women tend to find they store more body fat than men in general. Once they hit the 20% mark, they can likely start to see their ab outline. This can turn out to be further defined and even more obvious around the 16% mark. Many women can get under 14% body fat when they use the best training methods, because fat is stored around organs for protection, during child birth, especially.

The universal 10% body fat rule that most individuals/trainers endorse is perfect. You can go for more or less later, depending upon how you feel, and what seems right for you. We'll take a look at how we can achieve 10% body fat a little later in the title.

Due to how the body stores fat, some men (for example) might be around 12% total body fat with great visible abs, while others might need to get to around 8% body fat. Much of this depends on an individual's genetics and where their body might store stubborn fat. For a number of individuals, it's the legs, while others it's the arms, chest, or abs (belly region). We all store it in definitive places.

If the majority of your fat is stored on your stomach and you find you are lean in all other areas, you simply need to diet longer to get a great looking 6-pack. Regrettably, these are genetics and those we are unable to manipulate. With this in mind, we must be aware of what we already have, and what we must do to reach our goals. The training and diet schedules will give you some insight on this, soon.

## Ab Workouts vs. Conventional Workouts

We have already assumed you want a great 6-pack. I am actually going to advocate the stance that you minimize your ab workouts. While this might sound a little back to front and weird, it actually makes total sense when you come to understand that the principal restraining factor is your overall body fat, and not your abdominal muscles, overall.

As we have seen, you probably already have a great set of abs waiting for you. For this reason, we need to lose our body fat as efficiently and as quickly as possible.

To achieve this, we'll have to focus on workout routines which burn body fat as fast as possible. Unfortunately, because the core is a smaller group of muscles, in reality, it isn't very efficient in burning body fat. This is especially true, when compared to other exercise forms such as *Metabolic Resistance Training* (MRT) and *High Intensity Interval Training* (HIIT).

When we shift 80% of our focus (regime/time) onto these 2 styles of exercise, your body can burn fat up to 2-3 times faster, instead of trying to do it by performing lots of core/ab workouts. This increases the speed you are able to reach, and also the desired body fat level that is needed to reveal your 6-pack. As mentioned, once you start becoming lean and approach the point you are at your desired body fat level, you can now include actual core and ab-specific to stay shredded.

Heavy resistance training along with MRT and HIIT are far superior, because they burn a higher number of calories during the workout, while still boosting your metabolism for up to 48 hours, even once the session has finished. This, in turn, means you can lose weight quicker and continue burning fat even after you leave the gym.

If you enjoy training your abs, or you wish to train your core for added health benefits, this is fine, however, just do it 3 times a week as suggested. I'll explain this a little later in the title. And make sure it's not on your rest days.

## Eating to Promote Your 6-Pack

If your primary goal is to reduce your overall body fat level, then your diet will play a substantial role in this, too. By targeting your nutrition, you can efficiently burn body fat which then helps to reveal your abs and give you that fantastic 6-pack look. And one you can boost with exercise. When a healthy diet is combined with the above exercise methods (HIIT and resistance training), you will start to notice results really soon.

When you have a well-designed healthy weight loss/nutrition plan, you will see there are a few essential variables to master. Here is a quick overview:

**Protein:**

Protein is crucial when losing fat. Research shows it can help double weight loss while still protecting the hard-earned muscle you already have.

**Total Calories:**

Total calorie intake or energy balance or is also imperative. Initially, you must consume fewer calories than your body requires. This helps force it to burn your stored body fat. As a general rule for quick weight loss, I suggest you target around 11 to 12 calories per 1 lb. of overall body weight. For an individual weighing 200 lbs., this equates to 2200 – 2400 calories per day.

This is just a small amount of information pertaining to six packs, but I have a complete guide and formula in my title *"The six-pack formula"* it's completely Free to check it out. Click here

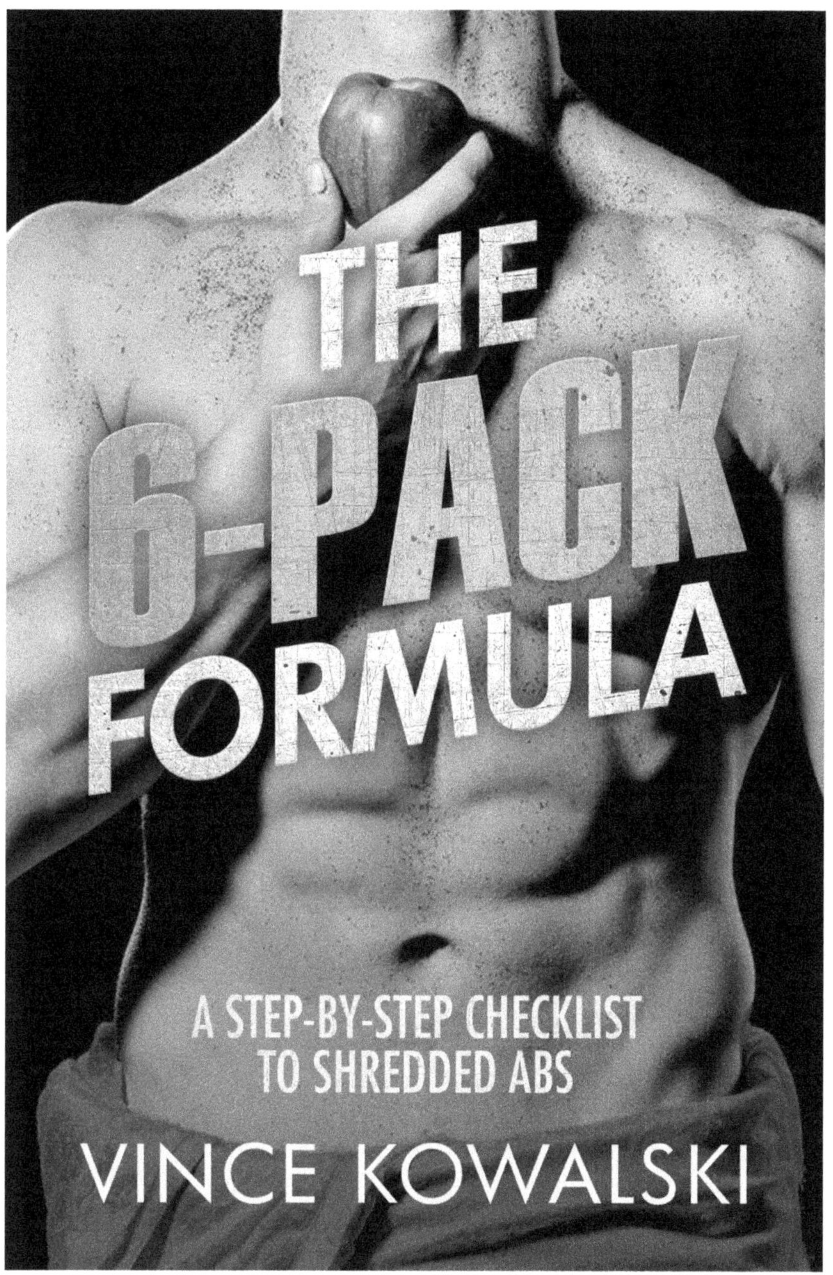
THE
6-PACK
FORMULA
A STEP-BY-STEP CHECKLIST
TO SHREDDED ABS
VINCE KOWALSKI

# AMAZING HERBS FOR BODYBUILDING

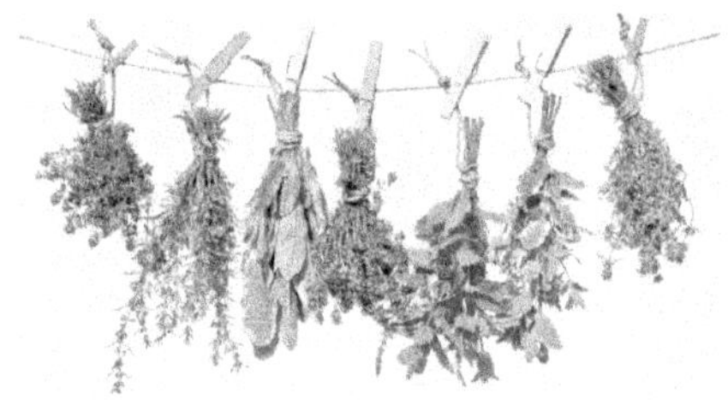

HERBS ARE USED AND ADDED TO FOOD TO IMPROVE FLAVOR. Today, around a third of all Americans partake in using herbal supplements in a way to help improve their overall health.

In fact, between 1994 and 1998, total sales of herbal supplements almost tripled and increased from 1.6 billion dollars to 4 billion dollars.

For quite a while, herbs were thought of as obsolete forms of medicine. They became pushed to the side in favor of drugs that were chemically produced and unnatural.

A vast number of people don't even know that half of the drugs which are in use today are man-made alternatives to natural, plant-derived substances. A good example being aspirin, which is little more than a chemical replicated salicin, an ingredient which comes from the bark of white willow trees.

Many drugs are now ineffective due to overuse and the constant alteration of pathogens with regard to the overuse of these drugs. The public is also becoming aware of the all-too-real side effects of many of these OTC (over-the-counter) and prescribed medicines.

Antacids being one of the most extensively used. These over-the-counter drugs are available, despite the fact that they can cause stomach irritation which, in turn, leads to individuals encountering worse indigestion. A vicious cycle.

Actually, medicines are no longer really concerned with averting complications or supporting a person's optimum health. The entire drug industry is built around making money. All you need to do is turn on the television and watch the advertisements for drugs as they flash onto the screen. It's as if they are just another candy bar. These days there is little difference, unfortunately.

Unfortunately, and on a global level, we have come to accept illness as unavoidable, and many people are more than happy to take an aspirin each day, instead of doing what is required for the prevention of a disease (or ailment) in the first place.

Herbs take a back seat and are very often not pursued, which is mostly because they are not as profitable, especially when compared to well-known drugs. This boils down to the fact that herbs reside in nature, and they can't be patented. It is much better to take a herb and improve health to avoid illness, rather than take a man-made drug (with side effects) when you are sick.

As a warning for your safety, and before I venture further into the uses of herbs. The content here doesn't have the intention of being the be-all and end-all of self-diagnosis. As with any medication, the same warning goes when taking herbs. You should always seek the assistance of a professional health care provider. This is to make sure that these herbs won't interfere with your current medication, or anything else that's added to your current lifestyle.

Because I am not a medical practitioner, this is being written as an information source for anyone who is interested in finding out more of the benefits that herbs can bring, and how they can be incorporated into a healthy lifestyle for regular people, or for athletic improvement.

## What Are Herbs?

The term "herb" is defined as either of the following:

1.  A seed-bearing plant which doesn't have a woody stem and dies, going back to the ground once it has flowered.

1.  A plant with leaves, seeds or flowers which can be used for flavoring foods, perfumes or for medicinal purposes.

We will use the word "herb" for any plant-derived substance which can be used as a useful, medicinal aid. When you look at the numbers, there are (in the region of) 380,000 documented known types of plants, with more than a few hundred thousand still to be discovered. The potential for more beneficial herbs is still enormous, with some still being undiscovered.

At present, there are around 260,000 plants which are known as higher plants. These plants contain chlorophyll and create their energy using the process of photosynthesis. Each plant which comes from this higher plant group can be used for medicinal uses.

Unfortunately, the number of plants that have been studied for their medicinal properties is only around ten percent. With the speed of development around the Amazon rainforest region, more of these plants are destroyed, so, we might not be in a position to see the value of some plants.

Active ingredients in herbal supplements can come from one, or several of the plant parts. This can include the roots, fruits, bark, leaves, flowers, stems, and/or the seeds.

There are numbers of herbs which show pharmacological properties and range from targeted therapy on specific organs or they can be used as an overall tonic with complete influence on the body, overall.

There are also some herbs, such as ginseng, which is known as an adaptogen. This term "adaptogen" refers to a plant substance that is all natural and produces no adverse side effects, even when consumed in more-significant quantities or for extended periods of time.

As the name suggests, an adaptogen has an overall tonic effect on the human body. They aid in the adjustment of numerous types of broad-based stressors. This helps in the overall efficiency of the internal healing system to increase. They also help in neutralizing any effects of overtraining, while still promoting speedy recovery and wellness.

Personal allergies should also be kept in mind. It is not to say you have to worry about an allergy when seasoning with a fresh culinary herb like basil or thyme (a meager 1 percent of plants are known to be poisonous), you just need to careful of what you ingest, and how high the recommended dosage is.

## Purchasing Herbs & Preparation

It is wise to remember that some herbs are very safe when taken for short periods of time. However, they can become dangerous with long-term use. You should only use any herbal remedy (medicine) for as long as is required, while always adhering to the manufacturer's guidelines.

### Capsules and Tablets:

Two-thirds of all herb supplement sales are made in capsule and tablet form. It is common for dried herbs to be put in a capsule or tablet with the precise directions for usage and dosage on the product label. From time to time, there will be herbal extracts in liquid form within a capsule. The typical dosage for both is 2-3 tablets or, in the case of capsules, 2-3 times daily.

### Extracts/Tinctures:

Liquid herbal preparations are known as extracts, or more commonly known as tinctures. These are generally made by the soaking of herbs in a water and/or alcohol mixture.

These extracts frequently come in either a bottle form (with a dropper for measuring dosages), or a set number of vials which are set for one serving.

You should be aware that a good deal of homeopathic extracts are considerably stronger than regular ones, and should be used following advice from a certified, homeopathic specialist.

### Powders:

Dried herbs can also be ground into fine powders which are to be mixed with water (before swallowing) to be consumed. On many occasions, these drinks will have a bitter taste of the herb and can be sweetened with honey, or you can purchase empty gelatin capsules and enclose the powder by hand to bypass this aftertaste.

## Dried Herbs:

On many occasions, these herbs are sold in large, airtight containers in bulk. When at home, all your herbs should be stored in the same way. You should choose a cool dark area.

With these purchased bulk herbs, you can either fill gelatin capsules and swallow as required or brew them as a tea. One tablespoon of the herb in hot water is the most common dosage. Drink (any made tea) hot or store any leftovers in the refrigerator to be reheated later.

## Prepared Teas:

A vast number of dried herbs can be purchased in teabag form ready to be brewed like any other tea. The dissimilarity between any medicinal tea, and teas found in supermarkets, is the potency. An actual medicinal tea will pack more power and should only be consumed as directed.

## Creams and Ointments:

Many herbs are shown to be beneficial when used externally rather than internally. Herbal creams are used to reduce joint pain or in alleviating skin problems and irritations, like eczema.

In experience, these products work well and are generally free from adverse side effects. However, some creams and ointments contain many potent ingredients and should always be used as directed.

## Personal Care Products:

Soaps, lotions, deodorants, toothpaste, and other various products are also available. Being (usually) all-natural, and with some herbs added to increase beneficial properties which relate to the products usage.

These products are usually effective and offer excellent alternatives to common, chemical-filled, personal care products. This is especially the case when you know the adverse effects of chemical additives. They are vast and shocking, in many instances.

Popular Herbs: Ashwagandha:

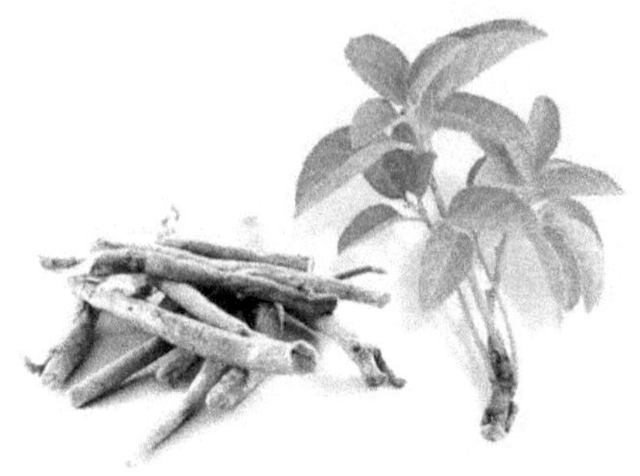

Ashwagandha (withania somnifera) is termed "Indian Ginseng," and this adaptogen helps with learning and memory. A study in India of fifty subjects who suffered from long-term lethargy and chronic fatigue were administered a tonic. One which contained eleven herbs with ashwagandha being one.

The patients had not responded to vitamin or mineral supplements and possessed no known illnesses. After consumption of the ashwagandha-based tonic for one month, the subjects reported a 45% improvement in mood. Additionally, blood-plasma proteins and their hemoglobin levels increased by quite a margin, which showed a general health improvement too.

Effects of ashwagandha (compared to ginseng) were measured to see the adaptogen qualities and anabolic differences. In a test involving test rats and mice, they were given an extract of ginseng, an ashwagandha extract, or saline for seven days.

On day eight of the study, the animals' endurance was measured by swimming. In the ginseng group, they swam for 62.55 minutes. The ashwagandha group swam for up to 82.14 minutes, while the saline group only swam for 35.34 minutes. This advocates that ashwagandha might be a stronger adaptogen than ginseng and also suggests that it might increase athletic endurance too.

## Cat's Claw:

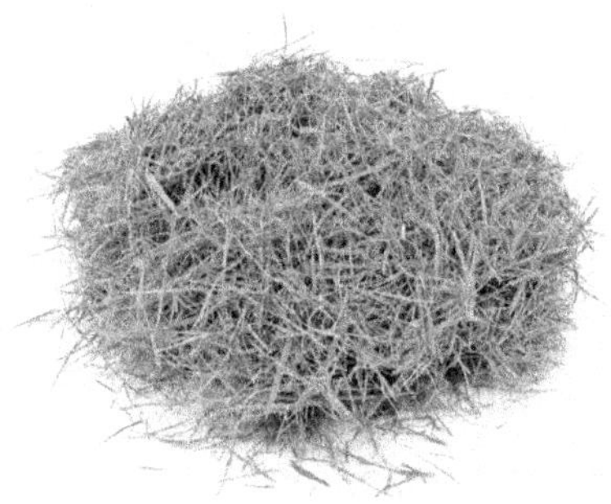

Cat's claw (uncaria tomentosa) is found in South America and is well known for its immune-boosting and anti-inflammatory benefits. Cat's claw can be used in treating many disorders related to the immune system, such as rheumatoid arthritis, Crohn's disease, herpes, and cancer.

It is also called "una de gato" and is commonly found in tincture or pill form. For quality, check supplements which are standardized to 15 percent polyphenols. Dosages of cat's claw are 500 to 1000 milligrams per day.

## Citrus Aurantium:

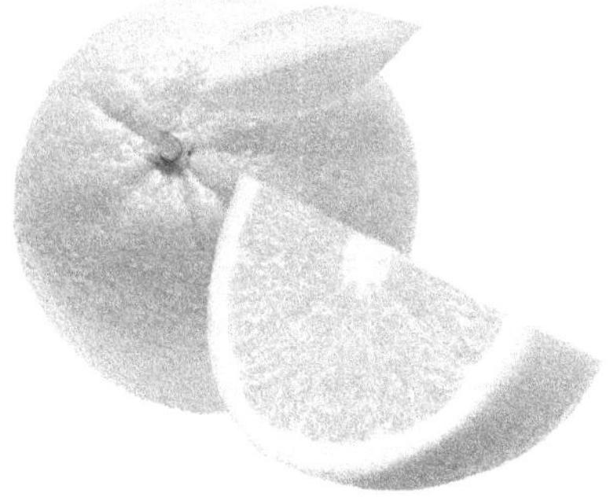

The unripe fruit of the green orange has been used in traditional

Chinese medicine for over 1000 years. Being taken to energize the body, with comparable effects of ephedrine. Citrus aurantium also improves digestion, circulation, and liver function.

Citrus aurantium contains a synephrine, a substance similar to ephedrine, and other thermogenics like caffeine and guarana, but without the side effects included.

Synephrine has been shown to be non-habit forming and doesn't act on the nervous system like ephedrine. Research shows it possesses antidepressant capabilities, while still increasing the cardiac output of the heart.

Check out products that provide 3-6 milligrams of synephrine.

**Echinacea:**

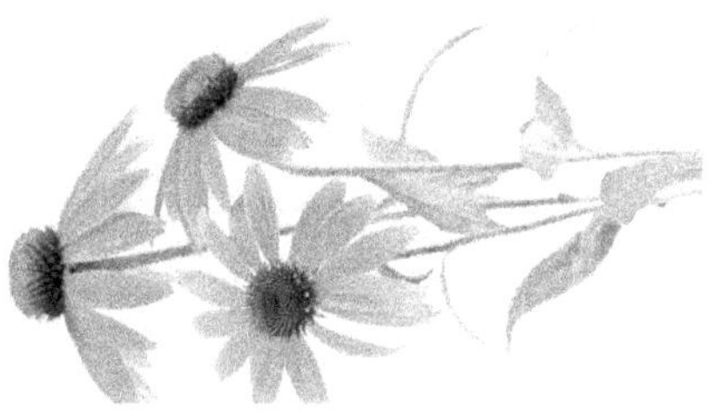

Native to North America, the American Indians use it more than any other herb, and it is the herb of choice for fighting colds, flu, infections, and a variety of other conditions.

Around 350 studies have investigated echinacea's clinical uses, with research concluding that echinacea has numerous immune-stimulating effects. According to European studies, echinacea can increase activity and the number of circulating immune system cells. It also enhances the production of natural immuno-active compounds, like interferon.

Nine species of echinacea exist, although only two of them (echinacea purpurea and echinacea angustifolia) have had an extensive study done on them. Check either of these out, for maximum benefits.

The recommended dosage is 200 to 400 milligrams, two to three times per day. Either on their own, or with other immune-enhancing herbs.

# 11

# THE WEEKLY TRAINING PROGRAM

I WOULD LIKE TO INTRODUCE AN EASY TO UNDERSTAND training program. It's very consistent and allows for the time needed in the healing, repair and growth of muscles. This is, therefore, utilized as a means for success and real, results-based achievement.

Always stay hydrated, focused, positive, and use the three pillars to keep you on track for the long haul. I always recommend adding great supplements to aid your body in its core nutrient processes as a necessity. Nutritional food is always great, but sometimes we need just a bit more to stay strong, energized, and give our bodies the sustenance needed to achieve awesome, long-term results.

Fundamental Core Weekly Training Program: (Add Required Reps)

**Workout #1**

Monday – Chest, Triceps and Abdominals

**Workout #2**

Tuesday – Shoulders, Legs and Abdominals

**Workout #3**

Wednesday – Back, Biceps and Abdominals

**Workout #4**

Thursday – Chest, Triceps and Abdominals

**Workout #5**

Friday – Shoulders, Legs and Abdominals

**Workout #6**

Saturday – Back, Biceps and Abdominals

**Additional Tips:**

- Abdominals are done every day, Monday through Friday.
- Every 3 days the whole body is done, over week everybody part is done twice.

**Workout #1 and Workout #4**

**Chest**

Bench Press - 3 sets of 10-12 reps

Incline Press - 3 sets of 10-12 reps

Flys - 3 sets of 10-12 reps

**Triceps**

Standing Triceps Extension with Barbell - 3 sets of 8-10 reps

Close Grip Bench Press - 3 sets of 10-12 reps

## Abdominals

Crunches, 4 sets of 25 repetitions


## Workout #2 and Workout #5

### Shoulders

Dumbbell Press - 3 sets of 8-10 reps

Military Press - 3 sets of 8-10 reps

Standing Lateral Raises - 3 sets of 8-10 reps

### Legs

Squats - 5 sets of 8-10 reps

Leg Extensions - 5 sets of 8-10 reps

Leg Curls - 5 sets of 8-10 reps

### Abdominals

Crunches, 4 sets of 25 repetitions


## Workout #3 and Workout #6

### Back

Lat Machine Pulldowns - 3 sets of 8-10 reps

Deadlifts - 5 sets of 8-10 reps

One-Arm Dumbbell Rows - 3 sets of 8-10 reps

**Biceps**

Seated Dumbbell Curls - 3 sets of 8-10 reps

Standing Barbell Rows - 3 sets of 8-10 reps

**Abdominals**

Crunches, 4 sets of 25 repetitions

12

---

# HOW TO EXECUTE EACH MAJOR EXERCISE

## Seated Dumbbell Curls

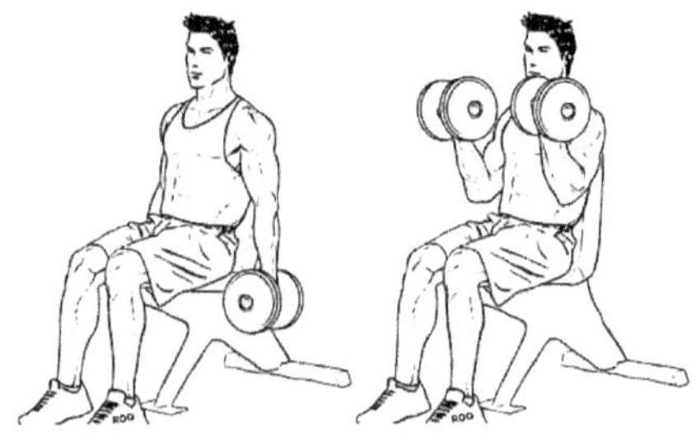

Sɪᴛ ᴡɪᴛʜ ᴀ ᴅᴜᴍʙʙᴇʟʟ ɪɴ ᴇᴀᴄʜ ʜᴀɴᴅ ᴀᴛ ᴀʀᴍ'ꜱ ʟᴇɴɢᴛʜ. Hᴏʟᴅ your elbows close to your body.

Turn your palms, so they are facing your body. This is the starting position.

Hold your upper arms stationary, then curl the weights and start twisting your wrists as the dumbbells pass your thighs.

The palms of your hands should face forward (toward you) at the end of the movement.

Make sure you contract the biceps as you exhale, and make sure only your forearms move.

Continue until your biceps are contracted entirely, and the dumbbells are at shoulder level. Hold this position for a second to squeeze your biceps.

Slowly lower the dumbbells toward the start position as you inhale and rotate your wrists back. Do this so you face your palms to your body.

## Standing Barbell Rows

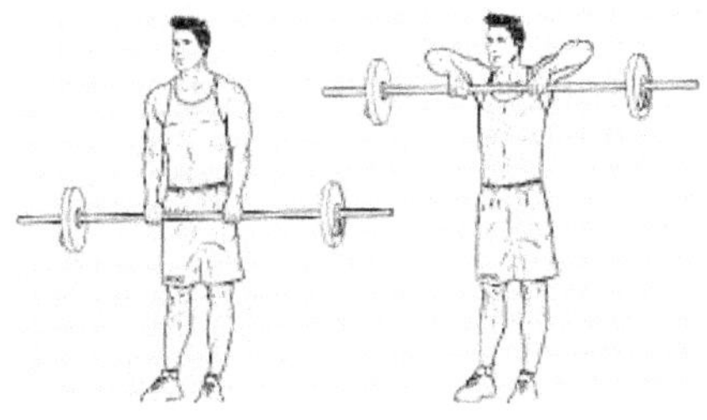

Walk to the bar. Stand with your feet halfway under the bar, and don't touch it with your shins. Stand medium width with your toes pointing outward.

Grab the bar a little wider than your shoulder width. Hold the bar low in your hands.

Bend your knees slightly. Keep them back so the bar will not hit them.

Raise your chest and straighten your back. Don't move the bar, drop your hips, or be tempted to pull your shoulder blades together.

Inhale deeply, hold it and lift the bar toward your lower chest. Lead with your elbows by pulling them to the side of your body toward the ceiling.

## Lat Machine Pulldowns

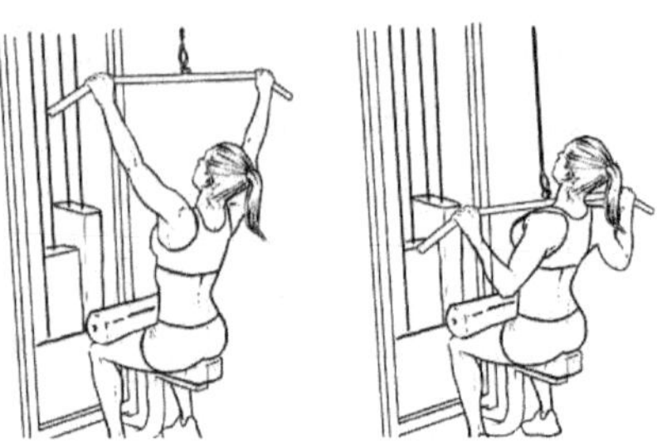

Sit at the equipment. Adjust the machine knee pad to fit your height. This prevents your body lifting when you pull.

Hold the bar with your palms facing forward. Your hands should be spaced wider than your shoulder width.

For medium grips - hands need to be placed equal to your shoulder width. A closed grip allows your hands to be placed so they are set narrower than your shoulder width.

Extend your arms in front of you holding the bar. Lean your torso back about 30 degrees. Create a curve in your lower back while sticking your chest out. This is your starting position.

As you exhale, pull the bar down until it touches your upper chest.

Squeeze your back muscles once you reach the full, contracted position.

Your upper body should remain stationary, and only your arms should move.

Your forearms do no other work apart from holding the bar, so do not pull the bar using your forearms.

After a second at the contracted position, inhale and gradually raise the bar back to the starting position. Do this as your arms become fully extended and your laterals are stretched entirely.

## Squats

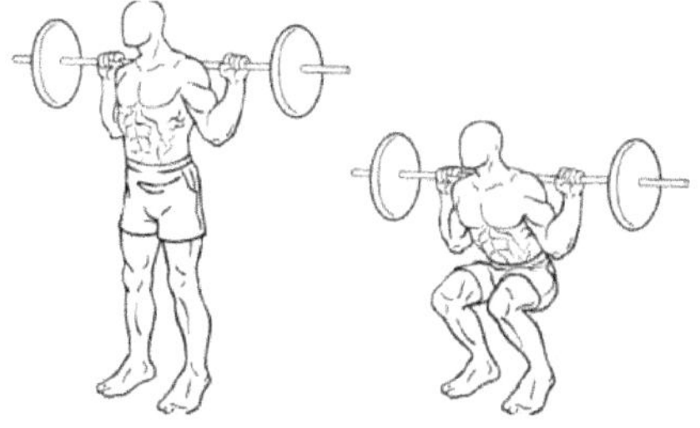

Stand with your feet shoulder-width apart. Turn your toes slightly outward. Pull in and tighten your lower abs, and keep your head and eyes facing forward.

Inhale as you slowly bend your knees while dropping your hips as you lower your body. Keep the heels of your feet flat on the floor.

As a counterbalance, hold your arms out in front of you at shoulder height.

At the bottom of the motion pause for a moment and exhale; then push back up to the starting position.

Keep your back as straight as possible during the lift to avoid any strain.

## One-Arm Dumbbell Rows

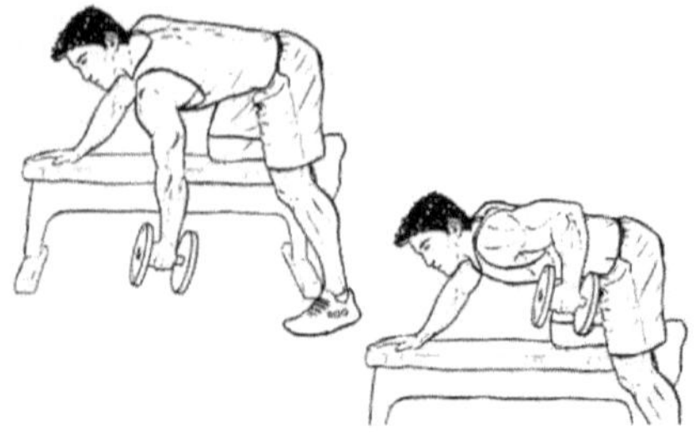

Place a dumbbell on each side of a flat bench.

Place your left leg at the end of the bench. Bend your torso till your upper body becomes parallel to the floor.

For support, place your left hand on the other end of the bench.

Use your right hand to pick up the dumbbell. The palm of your hand should face into your torso. This is the starting position.

Exhale and pull the dumbbell up to the side of your chest. Keep your upper arm close to the side of your body while you remain stationary.

Once your arm reaches the highest point toward your shoulder. Squeeze your back muscles.

Inhale as you lessen the resistance and lower the dumbbell straight down to the starting position.

Remember to switch sides and repeat with the other arm.


Leg Extensions

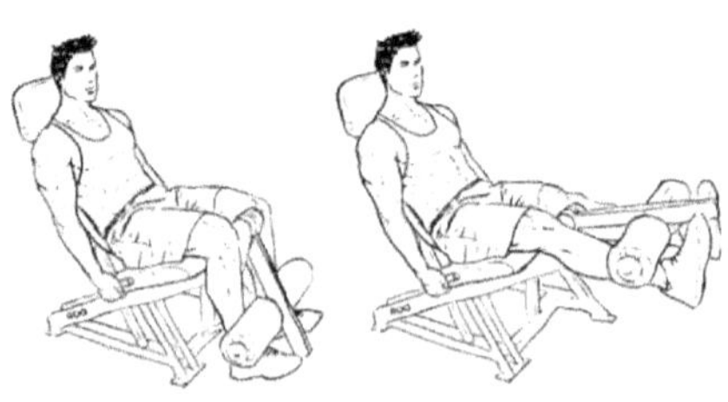

Select your lifting weight and sit on the machine. Place your legs under the pad (above your feet) pointing forward. Grab a hold of the sidebars.

Make sure that your legs are at a ninety-degree angle between your lower and upper leg.

Exhale and use your quadriceps; extend your legs to the maximum point in front of you.

Hold this position for a second.

Inhale and slowly lower the weight to the original start position.

## Leg Curls

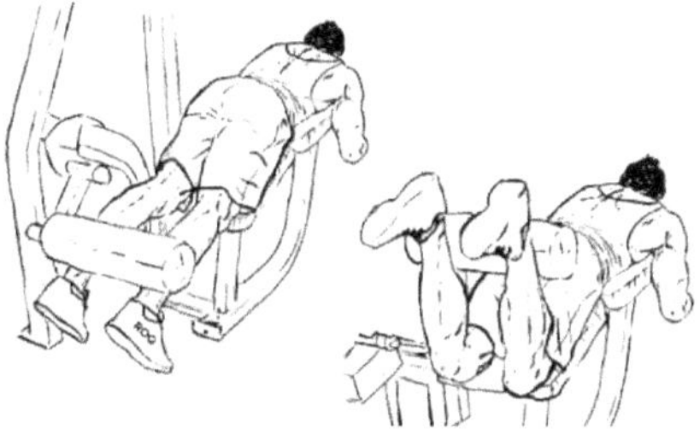

Sit with your back against the back-support pad and adjust the machine to fit your height.

Place your lower leg on top of the padded lever (a few inches under your calves).

Secure the lap pad against your thighs and above your knees.

Grip the side handles and pointing your toes straight.

Exhale; and bending your knees, pull down on the machine lever as far as possible under the back of your thighs.

Hold this position for a second. Inhale as you slowly return to the starting position.

## Dumbbell Press

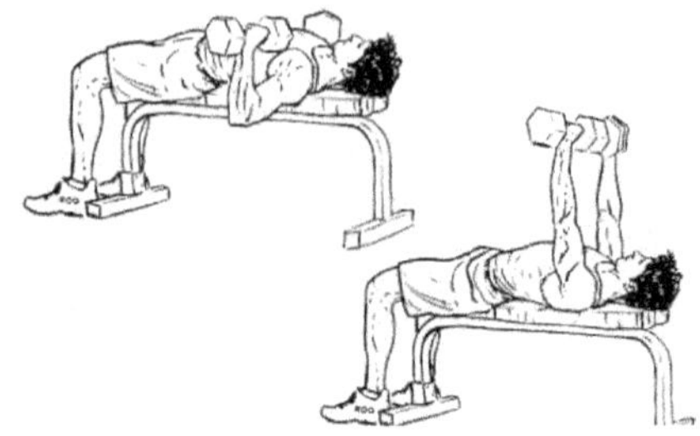

Lie on a flat bench with a dumbbell in each hand. The palms of your hands will be facing each other.

Once at shoulder width, rotate your wrists forward, so the palms of your hands are facing forward.

The dumbbells should be just to the sides of your chest, with your upper arms and forearms making a ninety-degree angle.

Exhale, and use your chest to push the dumbbells upward.

Lock your arms at the top of the lift and tighten your chest, then pause for a second.

Inhale and slowly lower the dumbbells.

Tip: Lowering the weight should take about twice as long as raising it.

## Military Press

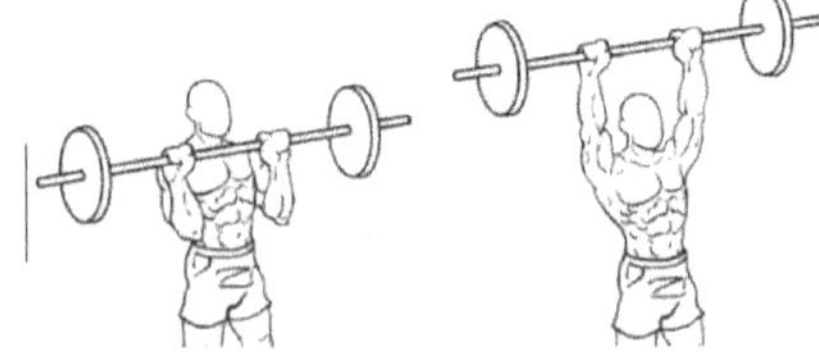

Position the barbell on the lifting rack to just below your shoulder height. Load the desired weights onto the bar.

Stand with your feet just wider than your shoulders.

Assume a shoulder-width stance (feet just wider than your shoulders) and place your hands at shoulder width. Now you grip on the bar with your palms facing toward you.

Step under the bar and raise it onto your collarbone while keeping your back straight and in a neutral position.

Take two steps back. Inhale and brace. Tuck your chin, and then press the bar above your head and lock your arms.

Pause for a second once your arms get to lockout.

Exhale and slowly reverse the movement while lowering the bar back to your chest.

Repeat for the desired number of repetitions and place the bar on the rack when finished. Use a partner to aid placement of equipment if needed.

## Standing Lateral Raises

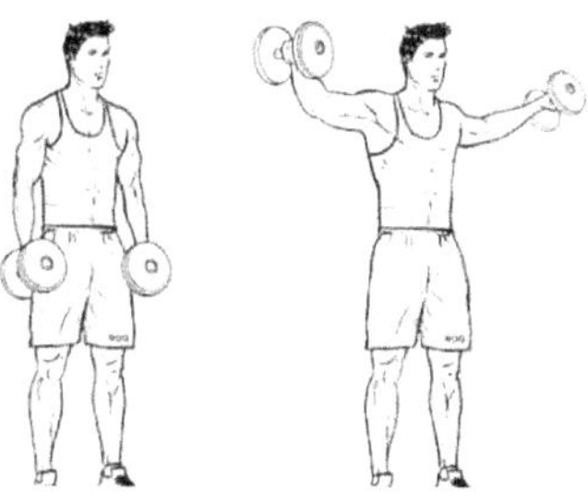

Pick a couple of dumbbells and stand with a straight back.

Hang dumbbells by your side at arm's length with your palms facing the sides of your body. This is your starting position.

While maintaining a straight and stationary torso position. Elevate the dumbbells from your sides with a slight bend on the elbow, and with the hands slightly tilted forward.

Exhale as you raise your arms until they are parallel to the floor and pointing sideways.

Once your arms are level, pause for a second.

Inhale as you slowly lower the dumbbells back to the starting position.

Repeat for the recommended amount of repetitions.

Bench Press

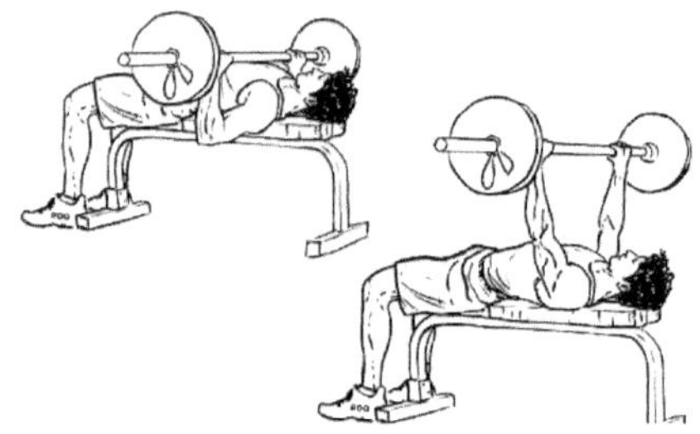

Lie or sit (depending upon equipment type). Use a medium width grip just slightly wider than your shoulders; create a ninety-degree angle on your elbows.

Raise the bar from the rack and hold it over your body with your arms locked. This is your starting position.

Inhale and slowly lower the bar until it touches the middle of your middle chest.

Pause for a second. Exhale as you raise the bar back to the starting position and lock in your arms.

Repeat the movement for the prescribed amount of repetitions.

When you are finished, place the bar back on the rack.

It is advisable to have the assistance of a spotter.

### Incline Press

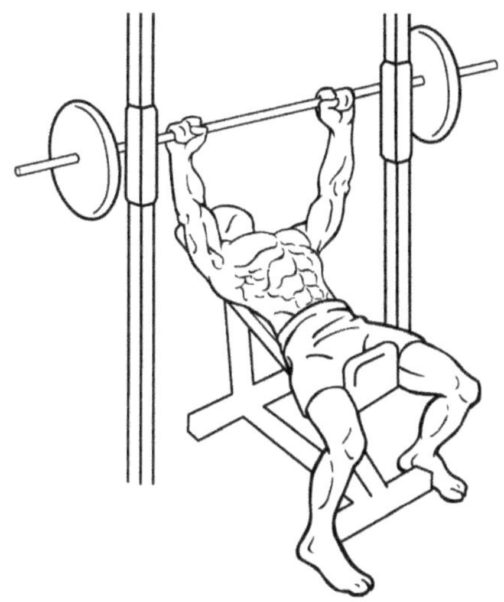

Load the bar to an appropriate weight for your training.

Adjust the seat to your height. The machine handles should be close to the top of your pectorals at the starting position.

Your chest and head should be up, and with your shoulder blades contracted together.

Exhale and push the handles forward by extending through the elbow.

Pause at the top for a second. Inhale as you slowly return the weight to just above the starting position.

Maintain tension on your muscles to prevent the weight resting back on the machine.

Complete your set of repetitions before letting the weight come to rest on the machine.


Flys

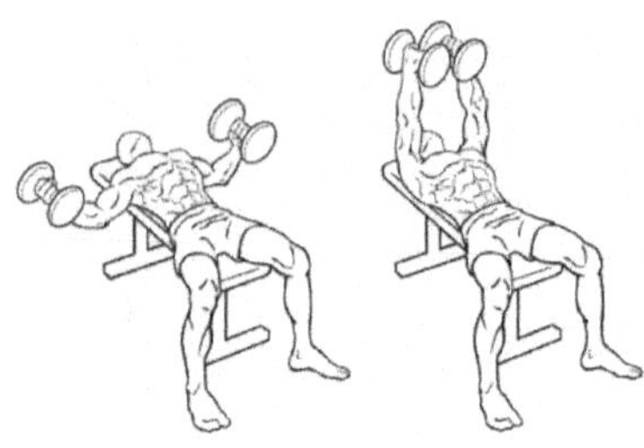

Sit on the machine and place your back flat on the support.

Take hold of the handles. Position your arms parallel to the floor and alter the machine to fit your size.

Exhale and pull the handles together in front of you as you tighten your chest in the middle.

When the handles are at their maximum, pause for a second holding the position.

Inhale and slowly return to the starting position. Use the resistance of the machine to stretch your chest muscles, as your hands return to your sides.

Repeat for the number of repetitions in your set. Remember to breathe.


Standing Triceps Extension with Barbell

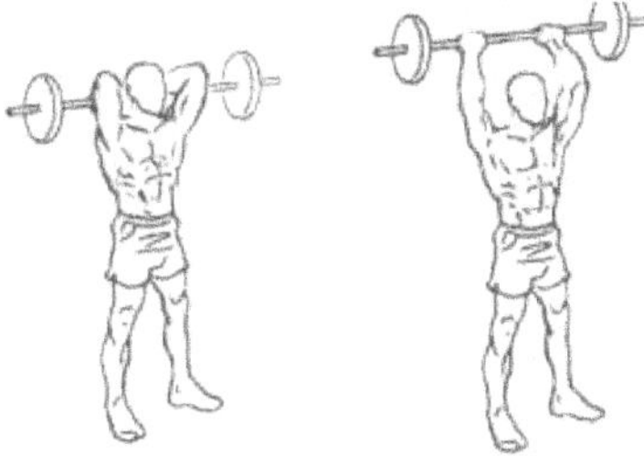

Stand holding a barbell with both hands. Your hands should be closer than shoulder width apart from each other.

Stand with your feet about shoulder-width apart.

Now raise the barbell above your head until your arms are fully extended.

Keep your upper arms close to the side of your head.

Lower the resistance in an arched motion behind your head until your forearms touch your biceps.

Your upper arms should remain still, and only your forearms should be moving. Breathe in as you perform this step.

Exhale and return to the starting position using your triceps to raise the barbell.

Repeat for the recommended number of repetitions in your set.

## Close Grip Bench Press

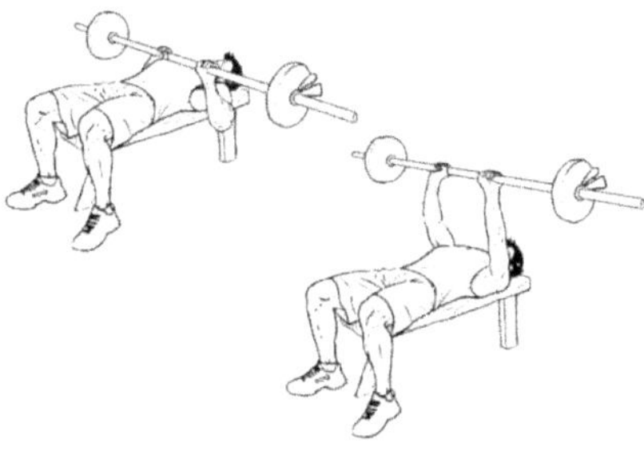

Lie on a flat bench. Using a closed grip, have your hands just inside your shoulder width.

Lift the bar from the rack and hold it straight above you with locked arms.

Inhale and slowly lower the bar until you feel it resting on your (middle) chest.

Pause for a second and then exhale as you push the bar back to the starting position. Do this using your triceps.

Lock your arms when you reach the limit. Pause and then repeat for the prescribed number of repetitions.

When you are done, place the bar back on the rack. Have a spotter during repetitions.

IN CONCLUSION

I'd like to thank you for taking the time to make your physique amazing! I know that you'll succeed if you put your time and effort in for the long-term. I'm so glad I could share my insights with you on a topic that I'm so passionate about. Additionally, I've done this so that you can meet your goals, without worrying about all the BS and marketplace hype that can be so confusing and disheartening these days.

If you follow the tips within this title, I know you'll be well on your way to getting the body you want. Your dream body! I congratulate you for allowing yourself to come this far. Please know that I am "virtually" cheering you on.

I wish you so much luck in the future, and I am sending all my prayers and positive thoughts to you in your weight training journey.

Thanks for spending your time with me here, God bless, always, *Vince.*

P.S. I truly believe in you!